Anxiety and Depression & Runners Handbook

As befitting its nature, it is presented without assurance regarding its prolonged validity or interim quality. Trademarks that are mentioned are done without written consent and can in no way be considered an endorsement from the trademark holder.

BONUS:

As promised, please use your link below to claim your 3 FREE Cookbooks on Health, Fitness & Dieting Instantly

tiny.cc/p5u27y

You can also share your link with your friends and families whom you think that can benefit from the cookbooks or you can forward them the link as a gift!

Table of Contents

Anxiety and Depression Cure:

Simple Workbook for Anxiety Relief. Stop Worrying and Overcome Depression Fast

Introduction

Thank you for purchasing, *"Anxiety and Depression Cure: Simple workbook for anxiety relief. Stop worrying and overcome depression fast."*

If you're reading this, it is most likely because you, or someone you know, is going through a tough time. By reading this book, you will gain a better understanding of how depression and anxiety work, how one can lead to the other, and how painful it can be to deal with both of these conditions.

When left untreated, both anxiety and depression can have devastating effects on those who suffer from these conditions. In some of the worst cases, people who have suffered from these conditions have gone as far as taking their own lives.

So, if you, or someone you know, is going through anything like this, this book will provide you with the information you need in order to seek help and get the right treatment. So, treatment will not only stop these conditions from worsening, but it will also help reverse its effects.

Unfortunately, many folks who suffer from anxiety and depression are left to suffer in silence. Often, those afflicted by these conditions are afraid to speak up and ask for help. Other times, the symptoms are so mild that they go undetected. That's why these conditions are almost never caught in their early stages.

In fact, seemingly bright and confident individuals are carrying this burden around with them. Even the strongest people you know may be dealing with these conditions.

Once, I heard a brilliant quote that said, "depression sets in when you have been strong for too long." Those were words that I could certainly identify with. They clearly sum up what most sufferers go through in their daily lives.

As such, this book is intended for those strong and brave people who are going through this themselves, or for those caring people that fear for the safety and health of someone they know. In either case, this book provides the guidelines for you to find the right course of action in dealing with anxiety and depression.

The first step is to acknowledge that you need help. Or in any event, to create a safe environment where the person you are concerned about can feel safe to open up. When that someone opens up, it might be messy, but they will have taken that critical first step on the part to recovery.

If this is you, one of those who are suffering in silence, then admitting you need help is hardly a sign of weakness. It is a sign that you are mature enough to understand that you have come to a point where you can't go at it alone anymore. And so, you are now ready to take that first step on the path to recovery.

In this book, we are going to talk about the basics of anxiety and depression, what they are, and how to spot them. This is very important since being able to recognize the warning signs early on can help save the life of a sufferer.

I mean it, literally.

When you are able to recognize the early warning signs, you will be able to seek treatment that will help you cope with the stress you are dealing with. That will cut out any chance of stress festering away until it becomes anxiety and eventually leads to depression.

Also, we will cover the ways in which you can get diagnosed for depression and the treatment options available to you or the person you are concerned about.

Next, we will look into ways which you can address anxiety and depression from home. That way, you can deal with the onset of any symptoms, as you spot them, and before they become a full-blown situation.

The most important thing to keep in mind on this journey is that you are not alone.

Even if there is no one around you, and you are reading this on the verge of a breakdown, you are not alone. There are people out there who are willing to help you and provide you with the reassurance you need. Some professionals specialize in helping folks who feel like all hope is lost.

Also, there are support groups filled with people who have gone through the same thing you are now going through. If you are concerned about someone else, you can invite them to such a group in order for them to see that this is not uncommon and that there are others just like them.

I would also like to encourage you to seek treatment from qualified healthcare professionals. It is absolutely vital that you, or the person you are concerned about, see a qualified healthcare professional who can provide the proper diagnosis and treatment options available.

Sure, there are times when anxiety and depression sufferers refuse to seek treatment. They may be in denial or simply too ashamed to seek help. This is why it is so important for you, or those you are concerned about, to understand that it is not your fault. Whatever the circumstances which lead you to feel this way, it is not your fault.

I would greatly urge you to act now. Don't wait a minute longer because the longer you wait, the worse things will get. By acting now, you will be able to get back on track or help those you are concerned about finding their way back to a healthy and productive life.

Unlike some conditions out there, anxiety and depression are perfectly treatable. Sure, there are medications which can help alleviate symptoms. But by treating the root cause of the issue, anxiety and depression can become a thing of the past.

So, let's start this discussion by looking into what anxiety and depression really are. I am sure that you will find a proper definition useful in getting into the proper frame of mind. When you see what these conditions really are, you will begin to understand the various options out there to address this situation once and for all.

Chapter 1: Definition of Anxiety and Depression?

In this chapter, we are going to be taking a closer look at what anxiety and depression are. We will be defining each term in addition to providing some insight into each condition.

When most people hear either one of these terms, they imagine some individual who can't keep it together. Hollywood films and television shows often depict depressed people as folks who are on the verge of suicide. And while untreated depression does lead to thoughts of suicide, that is not always the case. Also, anxiety is depicted as an unbearable feeling which leads sufferers to go through all kinds of unbearable situations such as lack of sleep, or uncontrollable shaking.

Of course, both of these conditions do have some of those symptoms associated with them; they are often prevalent in perfectly healthy people. These are folks who seemingly have everything together in life, but inside, are struggling with these conditions.

Other times, anxiety and depression get a hold of highly successful people who seem to have everything figured out. They are great at what they do, earn a decent living and are even the life of the party. However, they are struggling to keep their heads above water.

Then, some folks can't function anymore. These conditions have overrun them to a point where they cannot function as a regular person would. They cannot control their feelings to a point where even basic, daily activities can prove to become overwhelming.

But what is anxiety?

Anxiety is that uncontrollable, unshakable feeling of worry and concern about the future, what might happen or about things which are currently happening.

Sure, it's natural for everyone to feel nervous and anxious from time to time. Think about truly stressful situations such as taking a big test, or having to speak in front of a large audience. These are examples of situations which can cause anyone to lose sleep or even tremble with anticipation.

However, when the stressful situation is gone, then the person will be able to return to their normal condition. The stressful reaction dissipates and life goes back to normal.

For those who suffer from anxiety, life doesn't go back to normal. That's because there is no normal. There is only worry and anguish. This can lead the sufferer to lose sleep, become irritable and even experience physical symptoms such as digestive distress, skin rashes or overeating.

Thus, anxiety is generally a reaction to a stressful situation. Consequently, stress is the most important cause of anxiety though not the only one. While we will get into the causes of stress in a later chapter, it's worth noting that stress, or a stressful situation, will generally be the precursor to anxiety.

Often, the symptoms of anxiety are so mild that even the sufferer will have a hard time picking them up. These symptoms are often dismissed at just regular stress derived from working too much or having too many things to worry about.

Over time, stress builds up. Stress can build up to a point where the sufferer begins to manifest a condition called "burnout." In modern medicine, "burnout" is seen as a point in which the mind and body can no longer cope with chronic stress. Burnout is seen when the sufferer simply shuts down and begins to exhibit serious physical health concerns.

Nevertheless, burnout is just one physical manifestation of stress and anxiety. Since anxiety is predominantly mental and emotional, some sufferers may only present mild physical symptoms despite being emotionally distraught.

Fortunately, burnout can be treated with a combination of rest and medication. Anxiety, on the other hand, requires a much broader treatment, which may include medication, but almost always implies therapy. For some folks, their anxiety is just a condition they must live with for the rest of their lives and medication only helps alleviate the symptoms.

As for depression, this is, by far, one of the most debilitating mental and emotional conditions. Depression usually sets in as a result of chronic stress and/or untreated anxiety. For some folks, anxiety and depression work in tandem. For others, untreated anxiety leads to depression. Either way, depression can virtually destroy a person's life.

As with anxiety, depression sufferers aren't necessarily in bed all day wallowing about whatever it is that has caused these feelings. In fact, some of the most successful individuals you might meet are living with a condition known as "high functioning depression."

This type of depression is virtually impossible to detect as the sufferer does not exhibit some of the most traditional symptoms such as sadness and suicidal thoughts. So, depression can be defined as extreme feelings of despondency and dejection.

In short, depression is about feeling like there is nothing worth living for. It feels that life is not worth it anymore. When untreated, depression can lead to thought of suicide. And often, sufferers will act upon those thoughts if they do not receive the treatment they need.

Medically speaking, depression can be treated through a combination of medication and therapy. Upon diagnosis, a doctor may prescribe antidepressants and therapy. This combination usually leads to positive results though some depression sufferers may end up taking medication for the rest of their lives. However, prolonged exposure to antidepressants has serious side effects. So, this is why it is critical to address the root causes of the depression.

As I stated earlier, the symptoms of both anxiety and depression might be virtually undetectable. Nevertheless, there are warning signs which you need to keep an eye on. When these signs become all too frequent, you must determine if they are just the consequence of an especially stressful period or if it has become a pattern.

When the warning signs become evident, it is time for you to seek help, either for yourself, or the person you are concerned about. The sooner you are able to address these symptoms, the sooner you will be able to find a solution. The most important thing to keep in mind is that these conditions are treatable, and you can go back to being your old self.

Chapter 2: The Warning Signs Depression

When most folks think about anxiety and depression, they tend to think about a full-down, massive breakdown in which the sufferer is unable to function as a regular human being. These are often depicted in Hollywood films and television programs as people who cannot even get out of bed and take control of their own lives.

While this type of reaction can happen, especially when depression sets in at its most extreme levels, the fact of the matter is that most people go through their day-to-day lives functioning at a seemingly normal level.

In the previous chapter, I mentioned how high-functioning depression is a condition with which many successful people commonly live. They are able to function through their daily lives and routines, and apparently, not give off any signs that they are suffering from any kind of depression whatsoever.

Even in those cases, where successful people seem to have everything under control, there are warning signs that give away a person's internal emotional condition.

Let's start off with anxiety.

Anxiety is a debilitating condition which can hinder people from enjoying normal interaction with their surroundings.

Consider social anxiety.

When a person suffers from social anxiety, they may have trouble adapting and adjusting to the people around them. These sufferers may have troubling fitting into social groups like sports teams, classrooms, social clubs, churches, or any other place where groups of people gather.

Of course, there is a difference between a naturally shy person and a person who may be diagnosed with Social Anxiety Disorder. For naturally shy people, interacting with others on a regular basis may prove to be a challenging situation. For those who actually suffer from Social Anxiety Disorder, there is a deeper cause to their affliction. These causes may range from traumatic childhood events to physical issues in the brain. Nevertheless, anxiety, in all its forms, can keep a person from enjoying a healthy and productive life.

One of the most common factors which affect anxiety is stress.

Stress is a powerful force which can weaken a person's natural mental defenses to a point where they become excessively worried, or concerned, about what may happen to them.

Sure, there are logical reasons why a person may become overly anxious. For instance, if you are going through a difficult financial situation in which you have lost your job, need to pay the bills and are at risk of losing your home, the anxiety will definitely get a grip on you.

In this case, it is natural that a person has trouble sleeping, become irritable, lose appetite, or binge eat and gain weight, increase alcohol and drug consumption, engage is risk practices such a reckless driving, or even become isolated and reduce social interaction.

All of these symptoms, while concerning, point to a struggle with anxiety. Given the circumstances in which the stressful condition was created, all of these symptoms may go away when the individual's financial situation is solved. Then, they can get their life back on track through rest and possibly medication and therapy.

The symptoms which we have outlined begin in such a subtle manner that they are often imperceptible and go unnoticed. Many times, these symptoms are dismissed as, "being stressed out," or "going through a rough patch." But what ends up happening is that these feelings fester, and over time, can lead to debilitating anxiety, or depression.

In the previous chapter, we defined depression as having extreme feelings of dejection and despondency. This could not be more accurate.

Depression is a feeling in which the sufferer feels like all hope is lost. This is where suicidal thoughts find fertile soil. If untreated, depression may lead to somatization in which any number of physical ailments may develop. These physical ailments can range from migraine headaches to diabetes, heart disease and even autoimmune diseases such as lupus.

As you can see, depression is serious business.

Often, depression is seen as a psychological and mental disorder which requires medication as the first course of treatment. While there is no doubt that antidepressants such as Prozac, Zoloft or Paxil, which essentially inhibit certain chemical reactions in the brain, can be suitable options to help folks get back on their feet, the fact of the matter is that medication only treats the superficial ailments caused by depression.

In order to get to the root cause of depression, therapy is often required. With therapy, individuals can drill down and see what is fueling their feelings of dejection and despair.

Many times, chronic stress, which can lead to burnout, also leads to depression. When an individual is exposed to tremendous amounts of stress over prolonged periods of time, they can fall into a depressive condition in which their entire personality seems to morph completely.

Think of soldiers who go off to war.

A regular, healthy human being that is exposed to the large amounts of stress, such as war, may experience Post-Traumatic Stress Disease (PTSD). PTSD is a condition which arises from a singular, traumatic event that leaves an individual debilitated and unable to cope with everyday life. This condition is treatable, and recovery usually begins by removing the individual from the traumatic experience.

Now, imagine a soldier that has done several tours of duty in a war zone. This individual may be subjected to so much stress, that their entire personality morphs into someone else. They may go from being a kind, well-adjusted individual, to becoming violent and aggressive with the least amount of provocation.

This change may be perfectly obvious to those who have not seen this person for a while. But for the individuals themselves, spotting these behavioral changes is virtually impossible. That is how a person can descend into depression without even noticing it.

So, what can you do to spot depression in time?

You can be on the lookout for unusual behavioral changes such as emotional outbursts, unprovoked crying, or unusual euphoria. Yes, even euphoria and "joy" can become warning signs.

This type of behavior is evident in unruly children. When a child enters a depressive stage, they will often act out in violent and mischievous ways.

The reason for this lies in the fact that the individual is experiencing violent mood swings. And so, getting a grip on their emotions can become a hard task. That is why you must keep an eye on your loved ones especially when they are going through a hard time emotionally.

You must learn to interpret outburst and even destructive behavior as a cry for attention. This can be seen in excessive alcohol and drug consumption, reckless behavior such as driving and firearm use, or disengaging attitudes such as withdrawal and isolation.

If you are reading this and feel that some of these symptoms may apply to you, seek help at once. Find someone in whom you can confide. Ask them to take you to a proper healthcare professional who can provide you with alternatives on how to deal with your feelings. Please bear in mind that asking for help is not a sign of weakness. In fact, it takes a great deal of strength to admit you need help.

So, don't delay. Your family and loved ones will admire your courage. And, they will surely help you overcome what you are going through.

Chapter 3: What causes anxiety and depression?

In previous chapters, we have already touched upon the cause of anxiety and depression. We have discussed the triggers that most commonly induce anxiety and depression in individuals.

In this chapter, we will take a much closer look at the causes which can lead to anxiety and depression and how you can begin to understand why this is happening to you, or someone you know. The most important benefit of understanding the causes of anxiety and depression is that you will see that it is not the sufferer's fault, but rather, this person is a victim of circumstance.

So, let's get started with the causes of anxiety.

Causes of anxiety

Generally speaking, anxiety is mainly a psychological and emotional condition. While we have established that this condition can have physical effects on the sufferer, it mostly triggers a psychological and emotional response which can, in the most extreme cases, render a person unable to function normally in their regular, day-to-day lives.

Now, all of us experience anxiety to a greater, or lesser, extent. Allow me to elaborate.

Imagine you are a student and you are prepping for your final exams. There is a lot on the line, be it a passing grade, or a high grade which will allow you to get into the program of your choice at the school you most desire to enter.

So, you decide to put the pedal to the metal and buckle down on your schoolwork. Since you have a lot riding on your finals, the stress of getting good grades begins to get to you. You begin to have trouble sleeping, you may be losing your appetite, or binging on junk food, some individuals decide to take up smoking or drinking excessive amounts of coffee, or in some cases, show signs of irritability and overall bad mood.

Now, while this may seem like a "normal" reaction to high levels of stress, the person would go back to their normal behavioral patterns once finals are over and the stressful situation has been removed from the life of this individual. After a period of rest and recovery, the person goes back to their usual way of life having learned a valuable life lesson.

This type of reaction to anxiety caused by a significantly stressful situation is quite common and should not be a cause for alarm.

But what if this anxious behavioral pattern becomes all too common?

This is why it is important to differentiate one type of anxiety from another.

Anxiety due to a heavy course load is one thing, but it's another completely different thing to shut yourself off from the world because you cannot establish relationships with other types.

As such, the five most common types of anxiety are as follows:

1. General Anxiety Disorder
2. Obsessive-Compulsive Disorder
3. Panic Disorder
4. Post-Traumatic Stress Disorder
5. Social Anxiety Disorder

As you can see, we have already discussed these disorders to some extent. With the exception of PTSD, we have indicated how these types of anxiety all have their roots in some type of childhood trauma. Often, this trauma stems from some type of prolonged abusive or traumatic situation.

Think of situations in which children come from abusive homes, or backgrounds, in which they face neglect, physical harm, psychological and emotion distress, and even sexual abuse. While the most extreme cases of childhood trauma can lead to more serious conditions such as Dissociative Personality Disorder, prolonged exposure to trauma and stress can lead to the development of more generalized anxiety.

Of course, the development of anxiety does not necessarily have its roots in childhood. In fact, people who come from loving homes may develop some type anxiety disorder.

But how?

Well, in the case of PTSD, anxiety can stem from one, singular incident such as a car accident, the violent death of a loved one, or an incredibly stressful situation such as financial distress.

Anxiety can build up over time to a degree where the individual who suffers from prolonged exposure to stressful situations may not be able to fully recover once they have been extricated from the stressful environment which caused these feelings.

Think of people in high-stress profession such as stock trading.

The average lifespan of a Wall Street stock trader is about 10 years. Why?

Well, it's an incredibly stressful profession which demands constant attention. Most stock traders are plugged in for long hours with very few breaks in between. Since financial markets essentially run on 24 hours a day, stock traders may feel compelled to keep their foot on the gas even when they are officially off work.

In addition, the added burden that comes with the responsibility of managing large sums of money is hard enough. Most stock traders also face pressure from investors to make the best possible returns on the money invested. This leads them to make risky decisions which may or may not pay off in the end. The stress that comes from the uncertainty of a stock deal can keep a fella up for nights.

This is why alcohol and drug abuse has been seen among stock traders. These substances are used as coping mechanisms which end up costing individuals a lot more than then produce. Often, individuals who resort to substance abuse as a coping mechanism end up with a greater problem which is having to deal with addiction issues on top of their anxiety.

When this occurs, medication may be the only way to help an anxiety sufferer get back on track since the body, unfortunately, becomes used to those unusually high levels of stress.

In the end, the best course of action for people who find themselves in high-stress professions is to seek healthy coping mechanisms, such as mindfulness, which can ultimately help them deal with their anxiety in a much more productive manner thereby leading to a more well-adjusted mental condition.

Causes of depression

However, some folks end up being exposed to large amounts of stress for prolonged periods of time such as years on end. These folks may end up developing what is known as "chronic stress." Chronic stress, given that it is a "chronic" condition may never fully dissipate. As such, chronic stress is not the type of condition which will go away after a week on the beach.

As a matter of fact, chronic stress often leads to burnout, a condition which is often a precursor to full-blown depression.

When burnout sets in, the sufferer finds themselves feeling constantly fatigued, sleep deprived, usually overeating, abusing substances such as alcohol, caffeine or drugs, and even resorting prescription medication abuse.

Burnout tends to be confused with depression and depression tends to be confused with burnout. There are times when doctors prescribe some antidepressants and a good vacation thinking that sufferers are just tired and need a break. This is a critical mistake since a depressed individual actually requires a lot more than just a break.

Therefore, understanding that the root cause of a person's depression may be related to burnout and chronic stress is the first step toward helping the sufferer get back on track.

Other times, depression as deep and profound emotional root. This could be the result of a traumatic experience such as the death of a loved one. This is especially true when a person dies unexpectedly or passes on after a long bout with a terrible illness. The family members who are left behind are often burned out, emotionally distressed and in a deep state of sadness.

While it is perfectly normal to grieve over the death of a loved one, a profound sadness, which goes untreated, may end up becoming a full-blown depression. Once a full-blown depression sets in, the afflicted individual may become too affected to carry on with a normal life.

In addition, depression may take years to develop. As we have pointed out, chronic stress can be an underlying factor for depression. This is due to the fact that stress goes untreated, festers and then develops into a much deeper condition.

Often times, depression has a root in childhood. We have already indicated how abusive homes may lead individuals to develop some type of anxiety disorder. But it is also common to see adults who have come from abusive childhoods to end up developing some type of depression.

This type of depression can be categorized as "major depression" and can range from a debilitating condition in which the individual may need a combination of medication and therapy in order to cope with the situation or may need stronger treatment options such as rehab when there is drug or prescription medication abuse.

Then, there are other types of depression which may stem from purely physiological conditions such as Bipolar Disorder or Post-partum Depression. In both cases, the root causes are physiological and have more to the with the proper functioning of the brain than any psychological or emotional causes.

In the case of Bipolar Disorder, medication is almost always the only choice sufferers have. This enables them to rebalance the chemical composition in their brains and regain a great deal of normalcy in their daily functioning.

In the case of Post-partum Depression, the chemical and hormonal imbalances leftover from pregnancy may end up causing the most common symptoms such as sadness, fatigue, irritability and just a plain sense of melancholy. This is a condition which can be treated by a combination of both therapy and medication.

Depression is almost always a condition that never fully dissipates, even over time and with the right treatment. Unlike anxiety, which tends to show signs of recovery once the person has received treatment, depression can linger for years on end, and with frequent flare-ups.

For anyone who has gone through depression or has cared for someone who has dealt with the depression, will understand that there are "good days and bad days."

During "good days," the sufferer is often happy and in a good mood. During "bad days" the flare-ups may range from just regular moodiness to an all-out collapse. This is when you might see some folks going through periods of uncontrollable crying and sadness, to their body simply shutting off while they sleep for several hours on end.

This volatility in depressed people's moods is generally induced by certain "triggers." For instance, a depressed individual who is grieving over the loss of a loved one may experience a trigger when they come into contact with certain memories, places or objects. Therefore, it is vital to learn to recognize these triggers and avoid them as much as possible.

When depression is a purely, physiological condition, the sufferer needs to follow their doctor's instructions carefully, take their medication (if prescribed) and maintain a generally healthy and balanced lifestyle.

This last point is very important since the onset of a flare-up can happen at any time. Thus, it is important for the individual to recognize their triggers and act accordingly when symptoms are imminent.

In such cases, when the sufferer is well aware of the triggers which active flare-ups, it's important for them to be able to count on family and friends who can support them while they deal with the onset of negative feelings. This is especially true when the sufferer is exhibiting suicidal thoughts and tendencies.

In those cases, these individuals need constant monitoring. Otherwise, they may end up setting of a trigger which may lead to them acting upon such harmful thoughts. This is why I advocate the families and friends of depressed individuals to build communication and trust so that they are able to support and assist the depressed individual whenever they need to.

Unfortunately, those who suffer in silence lack this type of support. And many times, friends and family learn about the truth until after it's too late. That is why it is of the utmost importance that depressed individuals seek help as soon as possible. It may very well save their lives.

Chapter 4: What's Next After Diagnosis?

At this point, we have discussed causes of anxiety and depression, as well as, the symptoms which can be evidenced in people with either one of these conditions.

We have also stressed the importance of seeking help upon the realization that you, or someone you know, might have this condition. This is the hardest part: admitting that you need help and then looking for it.

If you are trying to reach someone who is being afflicted by this condition, it can seem virtually impossible to get through to them. Sufferers may even say they want help, but when it actually comes down to going in for diagnosis and treatment, you may encounter resistance.

In such cases, short of literally dragging someone to the doctor's office, there isn't much you can do to *force* someone to seek help. I used the term "force" since you really can't force anyone to seek help. This is something that each individual must really want.
Of course, there are cases when you must act in this manner. For instance, you might in the case of someone who is a danger to themselves. In which case, you need to step in right away before they hurt themselves.

Short of such a case, the ideal scenario would be to have the afflicted individual become aware that they need help and that there are healthcare professionals out there who are qualified in providing them with the help and support they need in order to get better.

So, the first step begins with admitting that you need help. When you are able to admit that you need help, you can then go out and seek it.

Generally speaking, you can go to your primary care physician who would be ready to provide you with immediate treatment. This could be in the form of medication which can help treat the most immediate symptoms such as insomnia, or mild antidepressants. At that point, your primary care physician would most likely refer you to a psychiatrist who can then begin a series of tests in order to determine if you, or the person you are caring for, indeed has a condition like depression or anxiety.

If you happen to find yourself having serious suicidal thoughts, or if the person you are caring for is showing serious signs of harming themselves, you may choose to take them into the emergency room. In this case, the most immediate course of treatment would be medication. This medication would most likely be a course in antidepressants or even a solid dose of sleeping pills.

Now, whether you visit the doctor on your own accord, or through an emergency room visit, a psychiatrist would most likely become involved in providing you with an official diagnosis. Other times, you may be referred to a neurologist to determine if there might be a physiological condition afflicting the individual. That evaluation may lead to a course of medication designed specifically for the condition affecting the individual.

If the cause is determined to be psychological and/or emotional, medication would be followed up with therapy and counseling. In this case, therapy and counseling are intended to help the individual understand why they feel the way they do and find positive ways of coping with depression or anxiety.

Now, an official depression or anxiety diagnosis is by no means a stigma. Unfortunately, there is a high degree of ignorance surrounding mental health issues. In mainstream society, people who suffer from depression or anxiety are seen as weak and unable to cope with life. This is why many choose to suffer in silence and try to deal with things on their own.

Granted, some individuals show a tremendous amount of fortitude and manage to pull through on their own. But there is also an equal number of individuals who do not manage to pull through and end up harming themselves. Sadly, some of these cases end up in tragedy such as suicide.

A positive depression or anxiety diagnosis is not a life sentence either. Sure, the severity of the condition may leave a person dependent on medication for the rest of their lives. This is something that must not be ruled out. Conversely, it must not be ruled out that with medication and therapy, as well as, other treatment options, an individual can regain a sense of normalcy in their lives and become free of their dependency on medication.

While becoming free from medication is the ideal scenario, it must be understood that reliance on medication may be the only effective treatment option. This is especially true in cases where individuals exhibit conditions such as Bipolar Disorder or severe cases of PTSD.

Perhaps the biggest factor in helping a person through depression and anxiety, especially in severe cases, is creating a loving and stable environment around them in which the sufferer feels safe and appreciated. This is especially true with children and teenagers.

When children and teenagers find themselves diagnosed with a condition such as depression or anxiety, their fears and insecurities come to the forefront. This will lead them to exhibit aggressive and erratic behavior which may stunt their development at a certain stage. This is why a loving environment would enable them to feel secure and allow them to process their feelings.

In the case of adults, having a loving and supportive environment is equally important. By surrounding the sufferer with a caring environment, they will begin to feel secure and may be willing to open up about how they feel. This is crucial when you consider how hard it can be for someone to show their vulnerability.

That is why a loving and supportive environment, in addition to medication and therapy, and other wellness techniques such as mindfulness, will become vital to helping you, or the person you care about, overcome this condition. I

So, I would encourage you to build a support network around yourself so that you can get the emotional support that you need in order to ensure you get the help you need, or that you are there to provide the love and support your loved ones need.

Chapter 5: How to Beat Anxiety and Depression

In previous chapters, we have discussed traditional treatment options for anxiety and depression. Traditional treatment options generally revolve around a combination of medication and therapy. This approach generally presents good results.

In fact, the combination of medication and therapy tends to be the best course of action, especially in cases when there is Major Depression, Bipolar Disorder, or even Social Anxiety Disorder. In these cases, medication is almost always the most effective treatment option as the symptoms are so severe that individuals may find themselves unable to function properly.

Furthermore, those cases in which individuals cannot take care of themselves, or even show signs of potentially hurting themselves, medication followed by therapy, usually in the form of one-on-one sessions or group counseling usually provides the best results.

But what about those cases in which symptoms are not as severe?

What about those cases in which folks are simply stressed out or a just blue?

When this happens, it is important to consider how you can address these issues without resorting to medication.

I always stress the fact that medication is not the only treatment option available. While medication may be the easiest course of treatment, it can also generate dependency in those folks who take it. Of course, dependency is not an ideal scenario as this may level to prescription drug abuse among other potential secondary effects of prolonged medication.

As we have also stated earlier, it is crucial to address the root causes of anxiety and depression. Often these conditions have psychological and emotional causes. When you are able to identify them, you can begin to address them in a holistic manner.

Other times, counseling may be the best way for you to address those root causes. You might find yourself in a support group in which similar folks can share their experiences in order to help you come to grips with what you are feeling.

In those cases, therapy and counseling provide tremendous benefits, particularly when considering that anxiety and depression in their initial stages are perfectly treatable and can lead the individual to make a full recovery without any lasting effects.

As I have stated earlier, untreated symptoms can fester until they become full-blown anxiety and depression. This may lead to individuals to become debilitated and unable to cope with the reality they are facing. When this happens, helping individuals recover and regain a sense of normalcy may prove to become incredibly difficult.

Consequently, catching these conditions as they begin becomes an imperative measure to be taken. So, please go back, if you must, to the chapter in which we discussed the early warning signs that you can look out for in yourself, or in someone you suspect may be going through this.

As such, we will be looking at an additional way to help overcome anxiety and depression that are not related to medication and therapy. These are ways in which you can find peace, solace, and comfort, especially when you are down in the dumps. In addition, these strategies can help you deal with your anxiety and depression proactively especially if you are already on medication and going to therapy.

Mindfulness and meditation

Mindfulness is the first step in helping anxiety and depression sufferers cope with their symptoms.

This practice involves meditation and relaxation techniques which can help you deal with the symptoms associated with anxiety and depression. In particular, these techniques can help when you feel the onset of symptoms that may lead to an anxiety attack or simply get your down.

The practice of mindfulness techniques will help you get a grip on your feelings by helping you develop a sense of introspection, that is, understand why you feel the way you do and recognize when symptoms, such as negative thoughts, are starting to get a hold of you.

So, you can begin with good, old-fashioned meditation.

Now, meditation isn't about sitting in a quiet garden, breathing, and repeating some mantra. Meditation is about listening to yourself, your thoughts and being able to examine your feelings from a third-party perspective. When you are able to achieve this, you will be able to figure out what triggers your feelings. For instance, it could be a repressed childhood memory, an object that reminds you of someone or visiting a place that sets off the recollection of an unpleasant experience.

As such, meditation, as a regular practice, will help you gain more control over your feelings and how you perceive yourself.

Here is a simple practice that I like to do especially when I am stressed out.

I like to find a quiet moment in my home and sit in my favorite chair. I know this can be extremely difficult to do especially if you have children running around the house all day. In fact, believe it or not, I have done this in my car when I cannot get peace anywhere else.

To start off, sit in your favorite chair and close your eyes. Place your hands on your lap and begin to breathe slowly. If you find that you are heaving, try to slow your breathing down by taking deep breaths. You can inhale, hold for three seconds and then exhale until you feel your lungs are empty. Then inhale again and hold.

While doing this, try to "listen" to yourself breathing. As you listen to your breathing, you will be bombarded by all kinds of thoughts. These thoughts may range from random stuff you have seen throughout the course of your day, to the insane and unpleasant thoughts that might be haunting you.

Try your best to not dwell on the bills, work, your boss, kids, car trouble, the loved ones that are gone and even the traumatic experiences you have gone through. They will come at you from all angles. But just let them pass. Watch them fly by. One after another. Imagine that you are just an observer watching a show. Concentrate on your breathing.

If you feel the anxiety building up, then pay attention to why you are feeling that way. Why are you feeling the way you do? What thoughts are triggering this reaction?

When you pay close attention to those feelings, you become more aware of your triggers.

Perhaps it was something someone said to you that hurt you deeply.

Perhaps it was something you saw which reminded you of an unpleasant, or even, traumatic experience.

Whatever the case, focus on why you are feeling the way you do. But don't stop breathing!

As the anxiety builds up, you may find yourself beginning to quicken your breath. That is where you need to slow things down. Slow your breathing down and focus on "listening" to each breath. As you do this, you will find yourself managing to get a hold of your thoughts and feelings.

Don't be afraid to face your thought. After all, they are just thoughts. As scary and daunting as they may be, they are just thoughts. They are in your head. So, you have nothing to be afraid of.

This practice is great especially for folks who have trouble sleeping. In fact, some folks like to listen to soft music while doing they are engaged in this exercise. Personally, I love soft piano music. This type of music is soothing, and it helps me concentrate better on my breathing.

As a matter of fact, this exercise works so well that I have fallen asleep quite often. As I said, it is great when you can't sleep because all sorts of thoughts are racing through your mind. I would encourage you to try this exercise when you are tired, and you can't sleep. You can lie in your bed, in a comfortable position and picture your thoughts, one by one, as they fly by the eyes of your mind. Soon, you will find yourself out like a light.

Being present

But mindfulness isn't just about meditation.

Mindfulness is a 24/7 activity which you do anywhere, anytime.

A great mindfulness exercise is to be "present." When you are present, you are not worrying about the past of the future. You are only concerned about the "here," and the "now." Sure, we can't erase the past with a giant magic marker, and we can't dismiss the future as we need to prepare as best we can. But being present means that, at this moment, there is nothing else around you. You are the only thing that exists. This will help you focus on what's going on at present and nothing else.

Being present is not about "forgetting" about the past and the future, it's about not concerning yourself with them. The past is done, and it's behind you while the future may not even happen; hence the trick!

You might be worried about something that may not even happen!

That is how being present is exactly the best way you can let go of the future.

Let go of the future?
Exactly!

When you stop focusing on what may or may not happen and prepare for anything that may come, you will put yourself in a great position to come out on top.

Consider this example:
Let's say that you are anxious about your health. You might be feeling very concerned about paying for your healthcare costs. So, you could decide to purchase some insurance for yourself and your family. In this way, you are covered in case anything happens. By having a proactive approach (getting insurance), you are covering your position in such a way that you won't have to worry about how you will pay for your bills since you already have coverage.

Now, this example may seem very simplistic, but it goes to show how something simple can set you up for something larger down the road.

The same goes for the past.

When you dwell on the past, you are dwelling on something you cannot change.

What does that mean?

Well, it means that there is no use in dwelling on something you have no control over. The past is done. So, there is nothing more to be. You are now in control of the present. This is why it is vitally important to live in the present; in the "here" and the "now." As you gain more practice and experience with controlling your current situation and surroundings, you will be able to make the most of the situations that are at hand. You will be able to relinquish control over things which you may not have any control over.

The case for a healthy diet and exercise

One commonly overlooked alternative is a healthy diet and regular exercise. This combination will help you feel much better about yourself. As you become healthier and fitter, you will get a boost to your self-esteem. As your self-esteem climbs, you will be able to focus more on continuing to improve yourself.

Furthermore, it is highly recommended that you moderate your intake of certain foods and drinks which may be harming you. For example, consumption of excessive amounts of caffeine, energy drinks and other stimulating substances can cause you to have momentary bursts of energy and euphoria but may leave you down in the dumps when the effects of the stimulants wear off.

In other cases, excessive consumption of junk food may lead you to binge eating. This is especially true when food is used as a coping mechanism. When this happens, you may find yourself consuming large amounts of food which is high in fat, cholesterol, sodium, and sugars. This can lead you to become obese and even trigger other health issues such as diabetes and heart disease, among other conditions.

In addition, it is also recommended that sufferers of depression and anxiety "clean up their act," that is, reduce, if not completely cut out, cigarettes, marijuana, or any other "recreational" use of drugs. Also, reducing, if not eliminating, alcohol consumption is ideal during the recovery process.

Just like you may become dependent on medication during your recovery, you may also become dependent on other substances. This is where it is important for you to take into account the need to get away from excessive consumption of certain substances.

As for exercise, exercising regularly is a great way to boost your mood. When you engage in any type of physical activity, your brain begins to release endorphins. This is the hormone that is associated with good feelings. That is why you tend to get a good vibe after you have finished your workout.

Also, trying your best to be fit will make you feel better about yourself. Consequently, when you feel good about yourself, you will be able to get a better handle on negative thoughts. As you become fitter and get into better shape, this will boost your mood, and your confidence, since you will be working on a better version of yourself. After all, who doesn't want to look fit and attractive?

Exercise should also be about engaging in activities which you enjoy. For instance, there is a sport that you enjoy playing such as basketball or soccer. So, when you take part in this sport, your mood will begin to improve since you are doing something you like.

I recall a friend that once told me about why he took up tennis. He was a high-power sales executive. He was constantly on the phone making deals and hardly had any type of slow down. He had a tough boss that demanded results. My friend was clearly one of the best at what he did, but after a while, he began to feel the effects of constant stress due to a high-paced life.

So, he took up tennis.

But tennis wasn't the first sport he had tried out. In fact, he had tried a number of sports and gave up on all of them.

Why?

Well, he told me how he was unable to concentrate on what he was doing. Thoughts about work and meeting targets would always come rushing to his mind. Consequently, he couldn't enjoy what he was doing as he was constantly worrying about the work he had left behind.

Then, he discovered tennis.
In his own words, he told me how hard it was for him to hit the ball. So, he really needed to focus and concentrate in order for him to hit the ball.

Voila! That did it.

He was able to find a sport in which he could concentrate fully and forget about the office. Perhaps his need to focus on concentrate on the ball was due to a lack and hand-eye coordination. But whatever it was, tennis became an outlet for him. Soon, he made buddies at his tennis club. This enabled him to get a grip on his anxiety and improve his overall health and wellbeing.

Therefore, I would encourage you to find a sport, or exercise routine, which can help you keep your mind off the stressors which are bearing down upon your mental health.

Aromatherapy

One very discreet way of keeping your negative thoughts in check can be through aromatherapy.

By surrounding yourself with pleasant scents, you are sending a positive signal to your brain. These pleasant scents will help you keep a positive vibe through your usual environment.

In particular, scents such as lavender and vanilla are great for helping folks relax. Nevertheless, I would encourage you to find your favorite scent and sprinkle around your surroundings. This could be in your office, your bedroom, and certainly in your car.

Also, burning incense is a great way of achieving that soothing effect that comes with pleasant scents. While you may not be able to burn incense everywhere you go, you can certainly keep some sticks handy at home and your office.

It has been shown that pleasant smells, even from perfume and cologne, can help reduce anxiety significantly. So, don't be skimpy on the pleasant scents. Get that perfume, or cologne, that you love. Ask your significant other to wear that scent you love. And don't forget to use essential oils to give your surroundings that extra soothing touch.

Don't forget about the visuals

It is amazing how visuals have a positive, and negative, impact on a person's mood. A cluttered and messy environment is often conducive to feeling even worse than you already do. In contrast, a neat and tidy situation will help you feel much better about yourself.

This is why it is highly recommended to keep a nice and tidy environment around you. This applies to both home and work. And, it also goes for cars and even wallets.

When you find yourself in a cluttered environment which may even be full of useless things, you will make it hard for yourself to find a safe place to call home. You may end up becoming anxious and stressed out because you can't find what you are looking for. In addition, a messy situation is almost always a precursor to depression.

So, take it upon yourself to keep your car, bedroom, office and living room as neat as you can. Now, I am not saying that you need to become obsessive about cleanliness. What I am saying is that a neat and tidy environment will do wonders to helping you feel much better about yourself.

So, it certainly pays for you to take the extra time to make sure that you have everything you need handy. By having everything in one spot, and knowing where everything is, you will be able to reduce anxiety by providing yourself with certainty and security.

Get a pet

Pets have been found to help reduce anxiety and depression.

In particular, it has been found that dogs can help anxious folks find a faithful companion who will help them find a balance. Something as simple as petting a dog can help reduce anxiety drastically. I have known folks who get a dog or cat, and just by playing with them, caressing them, and just having a pal around all the time, helps reduce anxiety by a significant margin.

Having pets can also help depressed folks get better by providing companionship especially when depressed folks suffer in silence.

In essence, what a pet does is that it provides unconditional companionship especially when the sufferer feels they are misunderstood or unjustly signaled out for whatever reason. Since pets cannot speak and behave much the same way humans do, sufferers find a companion who is not judgmental. Often pets, are there to provide solace during times of hardship.

While dogs and cats are the most common choices, other folks enjoy pet birds, fish, and even hamsters. The fact of the matter is that having a pet helps deflect negative energy into something more positive, such as taking care of a pet.

By being there for your pet, you too can get a sense of purpose. Other times, pets can become that impartial and attentive listener who is not going to pass judgment on the way you feel. They will kindly listen and give you all the love they are capable of giving.

One effective treatment option for anxiety, especially in children, is equine-assisted therapy. This type of therapy has been shown to help children relax and become more confident. It has proven to be especially effective with children who have a disability of some sort.

Horse have such a powerful effect on humans that the bond a persona may make with a horse, especially for children, will inspire confidence and security. This is what enables equine-assisted therapy to truly become effective. So, I would encourage you to look into this, especially if you have a child or teen who may be coping with anxiety or depression.

Seeking a higher power

There are times when seeking a higher power can help depressed folks kick the blues.

By engaging in spiritual activities, anxious or depressed individuals may find comfort and solace in a place of worship.

Generally speaking, seeking to connect with your spiritual self will allow you to connect with a deeper purpose for your life. After all, we all have a purpose in life. The challenge is trying to find out what it is.

This is where anxious and depressed individuals find a purpose in life. This enables them to kick the blues and channel their energy into seeking a deeper connection with the overall mission in life.

Seeking a higher power is especially forceful for depressed individuals. When a depressed person feels that there is a connection with a superior being, they feel that they are not alone. For those who have firm religious convictions, they can find comfort in knowing that their faith is capable of helping them get through whatever crisis they are going through.

Other times, churches provide a social group which can serve as a support group. I have personally found that prayer groups in churches really do make amazing miracles. It is the power of this collective energy which makes the sufferer feel confident and reassured. This positive energy becomes a new mindset for depressed and anxious folks.

One other significant strategy is not highlight passages in your book of worship. These passages should offer you consolation when you are down and serve as a reminder that there is always some higher power with you which can help you get through whatever you arc going through.

As your spiritual connection deepens, you will be well on your way to recovery.

A fresh start

In addition to everything we have highlighted in this chapter, a fresh start can prove to be just what the doctor ordered.

There are times when depression kicks due to a succession of adverse events. For example, you might lose your job, your house, your car, and even end up in divorce. Such a traumatic experience can certainly lead to serious anxiety and depression conditions.

So, as a complement to any, and all, of the options we have described in this chapter, what you may need is a fresh start. Often, this takes the form of moving to another city and starting over. This is typical when a specific geographical location makes it unbearable for the sufferer and sets off triggers continuously.

I have found it useful to wipe the slate clean at regular intervals.

For instance, I use each new month as a new opportunity to make something great of myself. This is especially true when you have a bad streak. The start of a new month can provide you with a psychological milestone whereby you can start over and put those negative experiences behind you.

The only time of year I would caution you to take care in starting over is New Year's. This occasion is a classic time when people, in general, get down in the dumps. For a person dealing with depression and anxiety, it may become tempting you make some New Year's resolutions which may or may not work out.

Nevertheless, a psychological signpost such as the start of a new year can provide you with the opportunity to push the "reset" button. Sure, it's not quite as easy as it sounds, but you can take the first step toward changing your situation and the way you feel about your surroundings.

Final thoughts

In this chapter, we discussed various ways in which you can address anxiety and depression from a completely different perspective that goes beyond therapy and medication. While this approach Is certainly effectively in helping most folks get their lives back on track, the implementation of any of the strategies discussed in this chapter will help sufferers get back on track and stay there.

So, if you are down in the dumps or someone you know is not feeling well, any of these tips will help boost their overall confidence and self-esteem. I am certain that these tips and techniques will go a long way toward ensuring that you, or your loved ones, will continue to be healthy and productive members of society.

Chapter 6: Understanding the Different Types of Depression

Thus far, we have discussed what depression is, its symptoms and treatment options. We have also touched upon the general definition of depression, that is, a profound state of dejection and despondency. Yet, there are specific types of depression, or division, into which this condition can be classified into.

So, in this chapter, we will be taking a closer look at each one of these divisions in order to gain a better understanding of the specific types of depression which can affect an individual and also learn about the difference between each type of depression.

Major depression

This first type of depression is known as "major depression." We have already discussed this type of depression at length. So, it's worth noting that a person may be diagnosed with this type of depression when they exhibit five or more of the symptoms associated with depression which are:

1. Chronic fatigue
2. Weight loss or gain
3. Trouble sleeping
4. Sleeping too much
5. Lack of focus
6. Loss of interest in pleasant activities
7. Withdrawal from social interaction
8. Suicidal thoughts
9. Feelings of guilt
10. Unusual irritability

These symptoms, while not exhaustive, are the hallmarks of major depression. As such, when a person consistently exhibits these symptoms, they may be diagnosed with major depression and provided with treatment options such as those already discussed in previous chapters.

Bipolar Disorder

Bipolar Disorder (BD), is considered to be a type of depression and is generally attributed to physiological causes. This condition is highlighted by violent mood swings which switch from opposite ends of the spectrum.

For example, a person with BD may be happily enjoying an activity and then suddenly become profoundly melancholy at the drop of a hat. Specific events generally trigger these type of mood swings.

Since physiological factors typically cause this condition, medication is almost always prescribed along with therapy in order for the sufferer to become familiar with the options available to them in terms of getting a handle on this condition.

Season Affective Disorder

Season Affective Disorder (SAD), is a type of depression which is associated with seasonal changes in weather patterns. It is attributed to a lack of sunshine and weather conditions associated with spring and summer. SAD is common in countries where there are harsh winters or significant rainfall.

Specifically, SAD is triggered by the persistence of weather conditions which limit a person's ability to enjoy common activities and limit their mobility. As such, they may become saddened by their inability to go out and enjoy their surroundings.

For this type of depression, a doctor may prescribe a mild antidepressant, though the use of techniques such as mindfulness and meditation is a great way of boosting mood and improving the sufferer's overall outlook in life.

Psychotic Depression

This type of depression contains, most, if not, all of the symptoms of major depression in addition to the following:

- Deep paranoia
- Hallucinations
- Delusions

These symptoms, in essence, transport the sufferer out of reality and into a state in which they feel, or believe, that something or someone is out to get them.

A person exhibiting these symptoms may receive treatment for other mental disorders such as Schizophrenia, thought a healthcare professional would be advised to dig deeper into the causes of psychotic behavior.

One very important note is that psychotic episodes are not necessarily accompanied by outburst of violence in which the sufferer intends to hurt themselves or others around them. These episodes may be highlighted by uncontrollable crying or sobbing, crippling feelings which render the sufferer unable to take care of themselves and serious thoughts of suicide.

Psychotic episodes are generally treated with sedatives in order to get the sufferer under control. In addition, strong antidepressant, or antipsychotic medication may be administered.

Post-Partum Depression

This type of depression follows childbirth. It can affect women of all shapes and sizes and cannot be attributed to any kind of physiological or emotional predisposition. Since it is generally hormonal, doctors may choose to prescribe a hormone regulatory course of treatment as opposed to antidepressants.

Women who are going to Post-partum Depression are encouraged to seek counseling as a means of understanding that they are going through and how they can manage their feelings. This condition generally dissipates over time and may not require further treatment.

Care needs to be taken as untreated Post-partum Depression may fester and eventually develop into major depression.

Premenstrual Dysphoric Disorder (PMDD)

This type of depression can be evidenced prior to the beginning of a woman's period. Since it is hormonal, a doctor may prescribe a mild antidepressant, or even oral contraceptives in order to balance out the hormonal load in the sufferer's body. It is considered a mild condition though, as, with any type of depression, it should not be left untreated when symptoms persist.

Situational depression

Situational depression is not an official term, but it is commonly used to refer to a condition in which a person is afflicted by specific events or situation which may lead them to exhibit the signs of major depression.

For instance, this could be the case of individuals who are under a lot of stress at work, school or have been through a traumatic experience. Often, this may be related to PTSD and treated as such. Other times, a doctor may diagnose it as anxiety and prescribe therapy and counseling prior to going on medication.

The symptoms of situational depression generally subside once the sufferer is removed from the stressful event.

Atypical depression

This type of depression may be considered as such in individuals who don't have any apparent cause for depression and do not exhibit the majority of symptoms associated with major depression. For instance, they may exhibit one, or two, symptoms but do not show the signs of a full-blown major depression. As such, it is important to monitor this person's behavior since left untreated; atypical depression may devolve into a serious condition which may leave the sufferer in a far worse condition than initially anticipated.

To close off this chapter, I would like to encourage you to seek medical advice when you see that you, or someone you care for, are exhibiting one, or several, or these symptoms of a consistent basis. By being able to address them in time, you will be able to avoid a serious medical condition which may require prolonged medication and therapy. By seeking help, you can take the first step toward regaining a sense of normalcy in your everyday life.

Chapter 7: Alternative Remedies to Overcome Depression

Throughout this book, we have discussed the treatment options for anxiety and depression.

As indicated earlier, depression tends to be almost always treated with a course in medication. Prescription drugs generally treat the chemical reactions in the brain which cause the majority of symptoms associated with depression.

In addition, counseling and therapy are also prescribed in order to help sufferers get a better handle on their symptoms and what they can do in order to improve their overall outlook on life and the condition they are dealing with.

In this chapter, we will be looking at three ways in which you can utilize home remedies to help deal with symptoms of depression. It should be noted that these remedies, by no means, should replace the treatment provided by a healthcare professional. Nevertheless, these remedies can be used in tandem to help the sufferer deal with the symptoms associated with depression, especially in a proactive manner.

Massage therapy

When you think of massages, what comes to mind?

Exactly!

Relaxation.

Massage therapy is a great way of alleviating the onset of negative feelings associated with depression. As such, it is important for the sufferer to be aware of the onset of these feelings in order to seek help.

This type of therapy can be done in tandem, or even alone by massage and stimulating certain pressure points such as the soles of your feet.

In essence, massage therapy can be something as simple as a shoulder or foot rub when feelings begin to manifest themselves, or it can be a full-body massage.

This is where I have indicated that massage therapy can be used as a proactive approach.

How so?

Well, the sufferer may choose to attend regular massage sessions in which the massage therapist may focus on specific parts of the body, or just do a full-body massage. Either way, the massage therapist should be aware of the reason for the massage so that they may take this consideration into mind.

In addition, sufferers may seek back adjustments in order to alleviate pain which may also be derived from bad posture or pain derived from muscle spasms resulting from large amounts of stress and anxiety.

Massage treatment should be discussed with your doctor beforehand in order to understand and agree on the best options available to the sufferer and maximize the benefit derived from this type of treatment.

Herbal supplements

Herbal supplements, such as St. John's Wort, are widely believed to help with symptoms of depression though there is no conclusive scientific evidence supporting this notion. That is not to say that the consumption of herbal supplements is not recommended or ineffective. What that means is that herbal supplements may end up doing little to actually help the sufferer's condition.

This is why you must talk to your doctor first prior to taking any herbal supplements. Of course, herbal supplements rarely cause any type of interaction with traditional medication, but it is worth discussing as your doctor should be aware of any such decisions.

Now, taking herbal supplements as a proactive approach especially when you are not on medication may prove to be a viable option especially when you are going through prolonged periods of stress due to a high-stress job, school, or any other situation which may lead you to show some signs of depression-like symptoms.

Another herbal supplement which is widely believed to help reduce feelings of anxiety and promote good sleep is Valerian Root.
This supplement is readily available and can be taken regularly when a person finds themselves in a stressful situation or may be having trouble sleeping. In addition, it is believed to help promote overall wellness in depression sufferers.

As with St. John's Wort, you should discuss this supplementation with your doctor if you are on medication. If you are not under medication, then this supplement could be used to help you relax and unwind at the end of a stressful day.

Other indications for this supplement are that it may be taken throughout the day especially during stressful situations. I would advise you to take it at home first and see how your body reacts. That way, if you choose to take it at work or school, you can be ready for the reaction this will have on your body.

Don't forget about yoga

The last home remedy I would like to recommend is yoga.

Yoga and meditation generally go hand in hand, though meditation is generally a mental and emotional exercise while yoga is a purely physical exercise.

When you do yoga, the positions require you to focus your mind and body on how you need to mold your body in order to achieve such positions. This tends to take the mind away from the causes of stress, and negative thoughts, and focus on the exercises being done.

Some folks feel that yoga is better done in a group rather than alone. This could be a great way of finding a balance especially if you suffer from social anxiety.

Also, yoga is a great way to start off the day on a positive note. 30 to 45 minutes of yoga exercises can help you feel relaxed and much more comfortable with yourself and your surroundings. Therapists often prescribe yoga due to its relaxation effects on anxiety sufferers.

For depression sufferers, yoga can be a great way to get some exercise in without even having to leave the house. So, it is definitely an option worth looking into. There are plenty of yoga tutorials online. As such, you can do these routines from the comfort of your own home.

Yoga, combined with mindfulness and meditation, will help you connect with yourself at a much deeper level. Consequently, you will be able to find a balance between yourself and a deeper consciousness that surrounds.

I highly encourage you to give yoga a try. It is one of the few exercises that provides both physical and mental practice.

Chapter 8: Alternative Remedies to Overcome Anxiety

In the previous chapter, we looked at a series of remedies which you can put to use at home in order to help you overcome anxiety and feelings of sadness, along with physical symptoms.

In this chapter, we will be focusing on remedies which can help you deal with anxiety. While depression is a clinical condition that often requires medical attention in addition to medication, anxiety sufferers may not be at a point where they need medication; they just need to find the right balance in order to ensure that they are able to cope with the stress in their lives.

As such, this chapter focuses on what to do, as well as, what not to do. Therefore, it's worth keeping an eye on the remedies which you can put to use in order to help you regain a balance in your day-to-day life.

Ditch caffeine, cigarettes, alcohol, and sugar

In general, anxiety has its roots in psychological and emotional imbalances. When this happens, you may find yourself falling prey to large amounts of stress that come with specific jobs and careers or simply having to live with negative situations such as the death of a loved one, illness, financial distress among other stressful situation.

When this occurs, folks tend to resort to substance abuse as a coping mechanism. Substances abuse can be as mild as overdoing coffee while getting into more serious situations such as the consumption of narcotics and prescription drugs.

Thus, one of the first things I would encourage you to do is to look at your diet and see which elements may be fueling your anxiety. For instance, if you are consuming large amounts of alcohol, you could be predisposing yourself for anxiety.

Also, having a healthy and balanced diet is one of the best things you can do in order to ensure that you are not setting yourself up for further anxiety attacks. In particular, high sugar consumption can put you on edge.

As a matter of fact, one rather common cause of anxiety is withdrawal-like symptoms when folks consume a lesser amount than they are accustomed to a particular substance. For example, drinking less coffee than usual may trigger an anxiety attack. The same goes for sugar and cigarettes.

In the case of alcohol and narcotics, the withdrawal-type symptoms may be so severe that medical intervention may be required in order to stabilize the sufferer. In which case, on common course of action is to seek a rehab facility which specializes in treating anxiety derived from substance abuse.

However, if you just drink too much coffee, maybe have a bit too many sweets and may overdo alcohol once in a while, it would certainly be worth having you cut down significantly on it. Ideally, you would eliminate the consumption of these substances, but that may not always be possible. However, if you feel that you would be unable to get such a habit under control, then it would be best to seek medical attention and rid yourself of these potentially harmful substances.

Stock up on tea

Tea is a great home remedy which you can use to help you curb your anxiety.

While it is true that black tea contains caffeine, there are a host of herbal teas which do not — as such, drinking tea may be a perfect alternative to drinking coffee especially if you can't wrap your mind around switching to decaf.

Herbal teas such as green tea are packed with antioxidants which can help your body rid itself of toxic substances while providing you with elements to help fight off high blood pressure and even clear your liver of unwanted substances.

Other teas such as chamomile, peppermint, and lemon are tasty alternatives to regular black and green tea. Chamomile has anti-inflammatory properties which can help reduce overall inflammation in the body while helping you calm down especially after a stressful day.

Peppermint and lemon teas have been found to not only contain antioxidants but have also been widely used as a soothing agent especially after stressful and traumatic events. Since both peppermint and lemon are loaded with antioxidants and flavonoids, they make for ideal choices when looking to calm down and unwind. Also, you can drink them throughout the day and serve as an excellent alternative to coffee.

Finally, teas such as Gotu Kola and Valerian, when consumed regularly, may prove to be as beneficial as taking as herbal supplement or even consuming mild antidepressants. Naturally, the key here is to be consistent in your tea consumption.

Prayer

Earlier, we talked about having a closer relationship with a higher power. Regardless of whichever faith you may profess, being close to a higher power is an absolute need for all humans. We all need to engage our spiritual selves in such a way that we able to connect with a deeper, more profound part of ourselves.

This is where prayer can help you not only connect with that deeper part of yourself, but also help relieve those feelings of anguish which may attack you from time to time.

I have found that regular prayer is a great way to help relieve feelings of uneasiness and uncertainty. Now, there aren't any specific prayers or mantras here. You can take your holy book and find a passage which is especially comforting, or you can recite prayers which are specific to your faith.

I would also encourage you to speak with your spiritual guide so that they may provide you with some ways you can engage your faith further. I have known folks who find peace and solace at their local church while others find calm in prayer groups.

Therefore, engaging in regular prayer and worship are two simple but effective elements which you can do in the comfort of your home or a part of a larger community. In addition, that feeling of belonging to a larger community will help you feel at ease since you can be sure that there are others who care about you and wish you nothing but the best.

Chapter 9: Alternative Remedies to Overcome Depression?

Throughout this book, we have discussed the ways in which you can help yourself, or someone you know who may be battling with anxiety and depression. Whether you, yourself, are going through this, or whether you are caring for someone else, there are many things you can do to help them cope with what they are going through.

Perhaps the single most important thing you can do is let them know that they are not alone. The worst thing that can happen to someone who is battling with depression, in particular, is to find themselves alone and uncared for. When this happens, the feelings of despair and despondency will only heighten. This may lead to suicidal thoughts and even to acting upon them.

You can help others battling with these conditions by providing them with a safe and loving environment in which they can be themselves. This is especially important for children and teenagers. Feeling comforted and cared for has a powerful effect to alleviate any of the symptoms we have previously described.

This point ties into showing sufferers how much you care about them. Perhaps you may not fully understand what they are going through, but you may be able to understand that they need help and support.

Now, this can be challenging especially when the sufferer is in denial and doesn't believe they actually need any help. In such cases, you may be met with resistance and even rejection. Often, anxiety and depression sufferers aren't aware of what's wrong and may feel offended that you are bringing up the subject.

Then, there are those who are suffering in silence. These individuals may be crying out for help in subtle ways. So, it's up to you to pick up on those and just offer and friendly smile and a shoulder to lean on.

When you have become aware that a person may be in a severe depression, then the time to act may be very short. When sufferers fall into severe depression, they may be inclined to act upon the negative thoughts they get. By this time, it may be too late to do anything about it.

Nevertheless, you can act quickly and seek medical attention for your loved one. This may include checking them into a rehab facility or even taking a trip down to the emergency room. Whatever the case, you need to act quickly. In doing so, you can ensure the health and safety of your loved ones.

Another vital element in helping sufferers cope with their condition is education. You can help them learn more about their condition, what triggers it and how they can find ways to cope with it. Bear in mind that someone in the grasp of severe anxiety and depression may not be able to fully think for themselves. This is where your support is vital in helping them understand the options available to them and what may be the best course of action. This may include medication or natural home remedies.

In the event that you, yourself, have been through this path yourself, you have valuable experience which you can share with others who are suffering just like you once did. I have found it useful to acquaint myself with others who have been through the same experiences as I have. These similar experiences have allowed me to develop a deeper understanding of what anxiety and depression are, and how to cope with them.

You may choose to engage in counseling, support therapy groups or just lend a friendly ear to anyone who is need of a friend. In doing so, you are helping others learn to cope with their condition and become self-sufficient.

So, I would encourage you to find out which organization support anxiety and depression sufferers in your local communities. Often, these organizations are part of larger health associations, churches, or volunteer groups.

Nowadays, most schools offer counseling programs for kids and teens. They not only teach kids how to deal with what they are currently feeling, but also provide a proactive approach so that these conditions do not develop in younger generations. I am certain that kids and teens would be interested to hear your experience as they may be struggling with something similar themselves.

Finally, helping others cope with their struggles is not an easy task as it can be emotionally draining. I have often felt helpless when trying to reach people who simply do not want to listen. While you may have all the good intentions in the world, these folks just need time and space before they can react to your supportive efforts.

Of course, the only time I would agree with your acting in spite of someone's resistance is when it is clear they are a danger to others and themselves. This is especially important with members of your family or very close friends. You can bring their family on board and get them the help they need.

In the event that the family of a sufferer is unwilling to get someone the help they need, you can contact a local social worker or healthcare professional who can assist you in finding the proper channels to get depressed individuals the help they need. This can be especially challenging when underage children and teenagers are being neglected the help they need.

At the end of the day, it pays to do your homework before attempting to help others. Do your research online, read books such as this one, take classes, attend seminars; do whatever you can to improve your knowledge base as this will help you gain more insight as to what you can do to help others find the right path toward regaining a balanced life.

Bear in mind that this is no easy task. But your dedication and efforts in helping others will contribute greatly toward ensuring the health and wellbeing of those who are struggling to cope with debilitating conditions such as anxiety and depression.

Conclusion

Well, we have come to the end of this incredible path. It seems unbelievable that we have covered so much in such a short period of time.

In this book, we have gone over anxiety and depression, their causes and the ways in which you, or someone you care for, can deal with them.

We have established how medical attention is essential in helping anxiety and depression sufferer cope with the condition they are facing. Often, sufferers are perfectly willing to receive help though they may not even know where to begin. This is why understanding treatment options are essential in helping sufferers overcome their feelings.

The most important thing to bear in mind is that the safety and wellbeing of the sufferer is the main thing to keep in mind. This is why recognizing even the subtlest signs of trouble may serve to help a person who is suffering, especially those who are suffering in silence.

This is why education is the first step. With proper education, you can learn about ways in which you can help others deal with this condition.

The most important thing to keep in mind is that sufferers are not alone. Depression, in particular, can heighten feelings of abandonment and rejection. So, being able to help sufferers by lending a helping hand is as powerful as tactic as any medication.

Ultimately, I would encourage you to consult your doctor especially before trying out home remedies and other alternative therapies. This is especially important if you are taking medication as potential interactions with other medications may have adverse effects.

Also, it pays to look into groups and organizations which you can count on to provide you with support and attention when needed. By being part of a support group, you can find a great source of moral support.

In addition, there are great therapy and counseling programs which are run by volunteers. Often, these are folks who have been through the same situation you are currently going through. As such, they can offer help and insights which are relevant to those who have dealt with similar conditions.

And so, I would like to thank you for reading this book. I hope you have found it useful and informative. Above all, I hope that you have found ways in which you can help yourself, and those whom you know may be struggling with this condition.

Please bear in mind that depression and anxiety are not a sign of weakness. After all, would you label a cancer patient as being weak? The same goes for anxiety and depression sufferers. Anxiety and depression sufferers are regular folks who are simply going through a rough patch. This is why helping sufferers feel that these conditions are not worthy of stigma or shame is a vital step toward helping them seek the help they need in order to enter the path to recovery.

I would also like to thank you for showing concern for someone whom you know may be going through this situation. I hope you have found answers to your questions though I would encourage you to further your study and understanding of these conditions and how you can utilize the many options which are available to you.

If you are struggling with these conditions, then I hope you have also found answers to your questions herein. I would also encourage you to ask for help. Even if you are alone, you can seek folks who can provide you with help and attention in order to get back on track.

You have already taken the first step on your road to recovery.

The Novice Runner's Handbook:

A Comprehensive Guide to Get You Started as a Runner or Jogger

Introduction

Congratulations on purchasing *The Novice Runner's Handbook: A Comprehensive Guide to Get You Started as a Runner or Jogger* and thank you for doing so.

The following chapters will discuss how you can get started as a runner or a jogger, and they will provide a lot of information that will motivate you to get out there and start running. The book will start by explaining how taking up jogging can transform your life in more ways than you'd expect. It will then proceed to explain the art of running, and what you need to do to make sure that you become a great runner.

As you read on, you will discover ways to find time for your running sessions. You will learn the reasons why scientists and medical professionals encourage people to take up running. You will also discover ways to become a better runner by pushing past your boundaries and setting new records for yourself.

You will learn how to choose the proper attire for your running sessions, and you will discover how to create your own schedule as a runner and how to make incremental improvements as a runner. You will also discover why nutrition is important to runners, and what foods you should eat to improve your performance. Finally, you will discover ways to reduce your chances of getting injured, but you will also learn about common injuries among runners and ways to treat and manage those injuries.

There are many books out there in the market about running and jogging, so thank you for selecting this one. We have made every effort to ensure that this book is full of useful information that will help you achieve great things as a runner, so please enjoy!

Chapter 1: How Running Can Transform Your Life

Running is the most natural form of workout that you can take up. It's easy to do, and it doesn't require you to spend a lot of money buying complex equipment or paying for an expensive gym membership. Running is one of the few activities that can actually influence your life and transform it for the better.

Running will make you much healthier, and it will improve the quality of your life for a long time to come. By running a few times every week, you can get lots of health benefits. They say that an apple a day will keep the doctor away, but the truth is that running can do a much better job of accomplishing that.

Running will make you happier. Scientists now know that running causes certain chemical reactions that get rid of negative emotions and replace them with positive ones. We will be looking at the scientific explanation for this phenomenon later on in the book, but it's worth noting that running is a stress reliever for which you don't have to pay anything.

When you take up running, you also transform your character in the process. Running teaches you to be more accountable and to be more methodical in your approach to most things in life. Running is an intensive activity that demands a lot of discipline, but those who take it up and stick to it learn an important skill that applies to other aspects of their lives. When you learn to account for your running sessions, you also become more accountable in your job and in your personal life.

Running teaches you to be ambitious. When you start running as a beginner, you will become more fit with time, and you will be driven to conquer your own boundaries and become a better runner. This will have the effect of improving your self-esteem as well as your confidence in your own ability to accomplish many more things. With each mile that you run, you will be more convinced that you can do greater things. As you push your limits as a runner, you will also feel the need to do the same with everything else and that will help you achieve things that you never imagined you could.

Running also helps you turn into a better version of yourself. Once you take up running, you won't be the guy who spends countless hours watching videos online. You won't be the guy who is afraid of physically taxing tasks. You will be the runner who challenges his or her own limits every day. That positive effect will stay with you, and it will transform you into a new person, a person who conquers all things.

Running will turn you into an optimist. As you increase your capacity to run and as you break records that you have set for yourself, you will start having a more positive outlook on things. You will look back at what you thought you couldn't do a few weeks ago and compare it to what you have done, and you will realize that you are capable of so much more. That optimism will infect other aspects of your life. If there is a project at work that you thought you couldn't handle, you will now start thinking that maybe all you have to do is give it a try. If there were other personal goals that you were afraid to pursue, you will start looking at them from a brighter side. It won't be blind optimism either because your accomplishments as a runner will serve as a living proof that you can be much better than you originally thought.

Running will also change the way people perceive you. After you have been running for a while, people will start noticing that you are leaner, more energized, more jovial, and friendlier. The way people perceive you is important because it affects the way they treat you. Your colleagues at work will start showing you more respect. Your family members will start having more faith in you, and in the end, everyone is going to trust your judgment a lot more than they did before.

So, don't miss out on the opportunity to transform your life. Read on, and you will discover everything you need to know to become a great runner.

Chapter 2: Running Is an Art, Treat It Like One

Running seems easy and it comes naturally to all of us, but if you want to do it as a regular fitness activity, you have to treat it as an art form. That means that you have to be deliberate about how you run, and you need to be mindful of all the body parts that are involved in the process. That's the best way to ensure that you reap all the benefits of running, including increased muscle strength and higher cardiovascular endurance. Professional runners learn to take an artistic approach to running by paying attention to all the body parts and making sure that they are properly utilized.

Running involves lots of body parts, including the head, shoulder, arms, hands, torso, hips, knees, legs, and the feet. We will look at how each of these body parts should be positioned or used as you go through the running motions.

How to Position Your Head While Running

It's easy to assume that running is only about the lower half of the body, but the fact is that if you want to nail down the art of running, you need to evaluate the whole body, from top to bottom, starting with the head. First, as you run, remember that your head needs to be upright, and you need to gaze straight ahead. When you are running, you are naturally going to get tired, and you will be tempted to tilt your chin either upwards or downwards. You should keep the position of your head in mind throughout, and you should keep reminding yourself not to tilt your head.

If your gaze is focused right ahead, you will be able to maintain the correct posture, and this will be good for your neck. Your head needs to be aligned with your neck as well as your spine. When you start running, especially when you are going fast, you are naturally going to feel the urge to put your head slightly ahead of the rest of the body, which will ruin the alignment between your head, neck, and spine. If you want to check whether your head is positioned correctly during the run, try to conduct a mental check and see if your ears are perfectly in line with your shoulder. If they aren't, it means that you have leaned your head further ahead, and you should reposition it.

How to Position Your Shoulders as You Run

In our daily lives, we spend countless hours hunched over our computers, phones, or desks, so we are used to placing our shoulders in the wrong position. When you go jogging, you should be mindful of the position of your shoulders. Instead of hunching over, you should open up your shoulders. Try to pull the back, as if you are trying to push your shoulder blades closer together at the back. Runners are told to push their shoulders back and their chests forward because by doing so, they can significantly boost both their endurance and their speed. If you run in a hunched position, you will be much slower, and you will get tired much sooner.

Don't move your shoulders in the same way that you move your torso. One error many armature runners make is that they try to move each shoulder with its corresponding leg. The correct shoulder movement should be; if you step forward with your left leg, your right shoulder should move forward, and so your left shoulder should be at the back along with your right leg. The opposite is true when you step forward with your right leg. This concept seems a bit confusing especially when you are doing it for the first time, but with some practice, you will be able to perfect it.

How to Position Your Arms as You Run

The position and the movements of your arms can have big impacts on how fast you run and how soon you get tired from running. If you place your arms in the wrong position, they could feel heavy after a while, and they could slow you down. If you move your arms the wrong way, they could ruin your balance, and you will be spending a lot of energy trying to reestablish your balance throughout the run, so you will get tired pretty fast. To position your arms correctly, make sure that your lower arms are at a 90-degree angle from your torso. Also, while you move, ensure that the motion of your arms is limited to the area between your chin and your hips. Moving one's arms from the chin to the hips helps with propulsion of the body, and this can help you move forward much faster.

Your arms shouldn't be in a wide position. In fact, you should keep your elbows as close to the torso as possible. Many untrained runners tend to make their elbows point outwards while they are running. This is a bad thing because it means that your arms will be in a cross position relative to your body, and this will slow you down. By maintaining the correct arm position, you will be able to get the momentum that you need. To help you keep your arms in the right position, you should train yourself by imagining that there is a line that runs through the center of your body and trying as much as possible to keep your hands from crossing that imaginary line.

What to Do with Your Hands While Running

Make sure that your hands are relaxed as you run. It may seem minor, but it's extremely important, and it can make a lot of difference for your performance as a runner. You want to focus all the energy in your body towards running, and when you tighten your hands, you waste some of that energy. This tip is more important for professional athletes than it is for beginners who are trying to keep fit. If your main focus is to burn as much energy as possible, it may not be of much use to you, but if you want to participate in a race, say a half marathon in your area, you should absolutely keep it in mind.

In order to keep your hands relaxed, you can try to imagine that you have something brittle between your index finger and your ring finger, and then you can try to loosen your fingers so that you don't crush whatever it is that you are holding.

The Correct Form for Your Torso

Your torso is extremely important when you are running because it's your source of power. When we are involved in most strenuous activities, we tap into our core, which is essentially the lower part of the torso. In running, the importance of the core goes beyond just being the source of strength. It's also the location of your center of gravity. So, of all the body parts that we will discuss in this chapter, you should make torso training one of your highest priorities if you want to fully embrace the art of running.

To position your torso correctly, you should always keep your spine straight, and you should try to elongate it as you run. You will naturally find yourself trying to crunch your spine, but you should fight that urge. When your spine is straight and elongated, you will be able to take advantage of the elastic energy that is generated whenever you step on the ground, and this will help you move forward much faster. You should also try to tighten your core so that you can draw strength from it and maintain your balance. Try as much as possible to channel strength from the torso as you run, instead of only using the strength in your legs.

What to Do with Your Hips as You Run

While running, you should use your hips to lean into the run. You don't want to keep your hips totally upright because that can reduce the length of the steps that you take, and it can slow you down. Leaning forward can help you run faster, but you need to remember that the lean should emanate from the hips, and not the shoulders. Essentially, what that means is that as you move forward while running, the parts of your body from the head to the torso (i.e. the parts that are above the hips) should be a bit forward from the position of the hips. This will give you a room to use your hips as part of the Gluteus Maximus, and it will help you summon more power which you can then channel into each stride that you make. If you lean your upper body forward relative to the position of the hips and if you use the hip hinge to lean into your run, you will be able to utilize your glutes more efficiently, and this can make a lot of difference in terms of speed and endurance.

How to Position Your Knees While Running

As you run, you should try to make sure that your knees are aligned to the middle part of your feet. The idea is that every time one of your feet hits the pavement, it should be positioned right under the knee. Also while running over a route that is relatively flat, you want to avoid lifting your knees close to or past the 90 degree angle because that would force you to spend a lot of energy (again, this might be okay if you are running for fitness purposes, but you should use the correct form if you want to master the art of running).

While running, you will get tired, and you will be tempted to shuffle around instead of actually running (the term shuffling refers to an action where people run while barely lifting their feet off the ground). If you find yourself shuffling, you have to try lifting the knees a bit higher. This will ensure that your feet are off the ground for a slightly longer amount of time, so you will be in a better position to realign your knees to the middle part of your feet. It's a difficult thing to do while you are tired, but with some practice, you will get used to it. You also have to ensure that your knees stay directly ahead of your hips with each step. Make a mental note to avoid bowing out your knees or turning the knees inwards.

How to Use Your Legs While Running

First of all, it's important to understand that we all have different ways of using our legs while running. It would be wrong to assume that everyone's stride is the same. However, all runners should try to make their shins perpendicular to the ground as they step down with each stride. For the lower leg to hit the ground at a right angle, you have to get your step just right—if you tend to step with your heel, your shin will be at a forward angle from the ground, and if you tend to step with your toes, the shin will be at backward angle from the ground. Either way, those aren't the correct positions for runners. They'll make you more susceptible to injuries.

If your feet land on the ground while your shin is perpendicular, you will be able to synchronize the motion of all your leg joints, and you could use this to your advantage to propel you further. By landing your feet correctly, you will be making it possible for all your 3 leg joints to work in harmony as shock absorbers, and they'll be able to create enough energy to boost your next step.

What to Do with Your Feet

You can use your feet to step onto the ground however you want. But the important thing to remember is that you should use them to push off the ground as you begin the next stride. Don't just use your knees to lift your feet off the ground. Pushing off with your feet helps propel you further.

Even though it's okay to hit the ground with the part of the feet that you feel the most comfortable with, many experts agree that the ball of the foot is the optimal part for hitting the ground while running. That is because it's a hardened part with fewer brittle bones and no direct joints that could get injured. However, if you feel that you prefer to hit the ground with other parts of your feet, you could get safe shoes that will protect you from injury.

Chapter 3: Finding the Right Time for Your Running Sessions

You may have considered taking up jogging for a while, but it always felt like you just couldn't find the right time to do it. In many cases, the real reasons why we always think that we are too busy to exercise are that we lack the motivation to get started, we are afraid of starting something new, we associate exercise with pain, or we think the whole experience won't be enjoyable. The fact is that when you make something a priority, and when you are convinced that it is extremely important, you will always be able to move other things around and find the time to do it. Here is how you can find the right time for your running session:

Write Down a Running Plan

You may have noticed that when you put things down in writing, they become more real, and you feel a deeper urge to see them through. If you have been planning to go jogging for a while and you never seem to get around to doing it, you may be able to give yourself a nudge by writing down when and where you intend to do it. You can either write it in your journal or program it into your calendar. When you take a look at your schedule for that particular day, and you will see that there is a fixed time interval that you have allocated to jogging, and your natural reaction will be to start preparing yourself mentally for that session. When the time for the session finally comes around, you will be more likely to actually go out for a jog. If you fail to actually see it through, the fact that you have missed it is going to bug you, and you are going to feel the urge to make up for it. Scheduling the running session is effective because it takes all the excuses out of the equation, so there will be nothing left to hide behind.

Spend Less Time Staring at Screens

There are lots of studies that show that we tend to spend many hours watching videos, either on television, on our computers, or on our smartphones. A study conducted in the US found that the average adult spends 6 hours watching videos every day! That's really a lot of time. Now, you might not be one of those people who spend countless hours staring at the screen, but chances are that you at least spend a couple of hours every other day watching something. If you can find time to watch anything (with the exception of the news) then you definitely can find time for a run—all you have to do is sacrifice watching your program, and you can do this by learning to practice delayed gratification.

Make Running Part of Your Social Life

Part of the reason we keep postponing our running sessions is that it eats into our social plans. Nobody wants to sacrifice the time they spend hanging out with their friends in order to go for a run. But who says that socializing and running have to be competing interests? It's very much possible to turn your running sessions into social events. For starters, you can convince some of your friends to take up jogging so that instead of putting on calories together at the pub, you can lose them together at the running track. Now, when you first ask your friends to give up the fun stuff and take up running instead, that could make you a bit unpopular in your social circle, but chances are that they too have been wrestling with the idea of getting started on a workout program, and you may be surprised to find that you have a few disciples who are willing to join you right away.

Make Running a Morning Habit

If you want to turn running into a habit, you'll have an easier time doing it if you schedule it as part of your morning routine. Waking up a little bit earlier in order to fit a running session into your mornings won't be easy at first, but you will get used to it, and you may even start doing it on autopilot. The fact is that things tend to change a lot during the day, so it's easier for you to postpone a running session if you have scheduled it for the afternoon or for the evening. When you slot your session for the morning, there is almost zero chance that something else will come up and force you to reschedule. Also, running in the morning is advantageous because it boosts your energy for the whole day, and it increases your performance and productivity.

Delegate Some of Your Responsibilities

Make sure that your family, your partner, or your roommates understand that running is really important to you and that they have to chip in to make your plan work. If you have chores at home which are preventing you from finding the time to jog, you can delegate them to your kids (this will teach them some responsibility and give them an opportunity to earn an allowance). If you are the boss at work, have some of your underlings cover for you as you take an hour off every other day to squeeze in a running session.

Put a Treadmill in Front of the TV

If you try your best to find time for a run but you are unable to, it might be wise to invest in a treadmill. The advantage of having a treadmill is that it's very flexible. You can use it any time of day or even in the middle of the night. If you find that you are unable to give up your screen time, it might be possible to integrate your running session into that screen time by putting a treadmill in front of the television. Imagine getting home from work late in the evening after a day where you had to go into the office at the crack of dawn. The only time you have is that hour that you spend catching up on the day's news or watching your favorite late-night program before you finally go to bed. If that's all you've got, you still can make it work. Just place your treadmill in front of your TV and run along as you watch your program.

Chapter 4: The Scientific Benefits of Jogging

There is a reason why you keep hearing medical professionals telling people to run more often. There are lots of scientific benefits that come as a result of jogging. These benefits are spread across all facets of your life. You may be primarily running to become more fit, but without knowing it, you are actually improving your life in dozens of other ways. Here are some of the most important scientific benefits of running and jogging:

Running Contributes Towards Weight Loss and the Reduced Risk of Obesity

This benefit is kind of obvious, but it's still worth mentioning—running can help you lose weight, and it can reduce your chances of being obese. A person that weighs around 200 pounds may be able to burn over 800 calories by running for about one hour. That means that if you run on a regular basis, you may be able to lose a few pounds every month and that could be exactly what you need to stave off obesity. If you combine a healthy diet, running, and other forms of exercise, you could very well lose a lot of weight. Running is advantageous as a weight loss exercise because it has a high after-burn rate (this is where your body keep burning calories even after you are done working out).

Running Boosts Your Mental Acuity

There is a lot of scientific evidence out there that shows that running can increase your mental acuity and improve your brain's performance. In fact, people who jog on a regular basis tend to perform better than those who don't in memory tests. Neuroscientists believe that running actually promotes the generation of new nerve cells, which improves people's motor skills and general mental sharpness. There is also evidence that running can help stave off conditions that cause the decline of memory and other brain functions. If you run more in your youth, you will be less likely to get Alzheimer's disease and dementia when you are much older.

Running Can Help Relieve Stress

When you run, your body produces feel-good hormones which boost your mood and reduce stress and anxiety. Endorphins have been known to alleviate stress and reduce the risk of having migraines as well as tension headaches. When you run, your heart rate increases. That increase in heart rate has the effect of repairing the parts of the brain that have been adversely affected by stressful experiences. Also, psychologically speaking, when you run out in nature, you will be able to clear your brain, breath in some fresh air, and rid yourself of any stressful thoughts.

Running Is Linked to Reduced Risk of Cancer

There is some research that shows that running can reduce the risk of some forms of cancer. Studies have indicated that regular jogging (or even fast-paced walking) can lower the risk of breast cancer by about 14%. Additionally, there are more than 150 other studies out there that show that the risk of various types of cancer is reduced when people take up running and other types of exercises.

Running Protects You from Cardiovascular Diseases

You probably have heard about "heart run" marathons, or you have heard the surgeon general encouraging people to run more to reduce the risk of heart disease. Cardiovascular diseases are leading causes of death the world over, so don't assume that you won't be affected by them. One recent study showed that runners are 45% less likely to die as a result of cardiovascular diseases. Also, people who run regularly, even for less than ten minutes, can cut their risk of cardiovascular diseases by about a half.

Running Increases Your Level of Happiness

It may not seem so when you are in the middle of an intense running session, but running actually makes people happier, and there is scientific evidence to prove it. Studies have shown that exercise has the effect of relieving anxiety, alleviating depression, and reducing stress, all while energizing your body and making you more jovial. You have probably heard of the term "runner's high." It refers to a sense of euphoria that comes about due to the release of endorphins after you have been running for a while. When you are dealing with all kinds of stressful issues, including personal relationship problems, issues at work, etc., you may be able to improve your mood and regain your composure if you take some time to go out for a run.

Running Can Help Reduce Insomnia and Other Sleep-Related Problems

Are you having a difficult time going to sleep every night? Do you suffer from other sleep-related conditions? Well, according to scientific evidence, running has the effect of promoting your quality of sleep. First, if you run during the day, you will be more tired at night, and you will have an easier time falling asleep. When you are energized during the day as you work out, that energy tends to dissipate by the time you go to bed, so your body will be feeling the need to rejuvenate itself by resting. If you aren't invigorated during the day, the pent-up energy will still be in your body when you go to sleep, and that could be the cause of your insomnia. Sleep issues may also be a result of stress, and since running reduces stress, it could also contribute to better sleep in an indirect way.

Running Increases Your Life Expectancy

Running is considered one of the most effective ways to increase your lifespan and to help improve the quality of the life that you live. There are lots of studies that bear witness to that fact. One study out of Stanford University looked at data spanning two whole decades, and it found that people who run regularly live longer than those who don't. In fact, of all the people who participated in that study, 80% of those who were runners are still alive, while in the non-runner category, it's only 65% who are still alive. That is a huge difference that you shouldn't overlook. The next time you are out jogging, you should remember that you are actually running for your life.

Chapter 5: How to Push It to the Limit and Challenge Your Boundaries as a Runner

Just like any other fitness activity that you have to perform every day, running can become monotonous, and you can end up getting stuck in a rut and fail to improve or to push your boundaries. The fact is that many people pick up running as an activity, and they stay faithful to their routines, only to find that weeks or even months down the line, they haven't improved on their speed or their endurance. That's because, just like in any other activities, we can also get stuck inside our comfort zones as runners.

To grow as a runner, you must set goals that are achievable, and you must strive to make gradual improvements in relation to your speed and your endurance as the days go by. In this chapter, we will discuss tips and tricks that can help you challenge your boundaries as a runner so that you can achieve higher levels of fitness.

Learn How to Stay Positive During Your Runs

Your ability to push your own limits depends on your attitude. If you have a positive attitude, you will be able to get the mental fortitude to keep going even when your body is telling you to give up. There are lots of tips and tricks that are used by professional athletes and people who perform physically tasking activities. You can try them out one by one, and then, you can decide to adopt the ones that you believe suit you the best.

The first trick is to use positive mantras and affirmations as you run. You have to keep repeating a phrase in your head to keep yourself motivated during the entire run. The mantra that you select should be short, positive, and self-affirming. You can use phrases such as "yes I can" or "keep it on." You can customize your own mantra into something that you find inspiring. For example, you can take a section of your favorite quote about hard work or persistence and use it as your mantra. You need to coordinate your mantra chants with your breathing pattern so that it acts as a tempo that can help you pace yourself as you jog. If you have been running for a while, you will naturally develop a rhythmic breathing pattern. Try to repeat the mantra in your head between breaths and make a conscious effort to truly believe in the premise of your mantra. Before you know it, you will be running a little longer or a bit faster.

The second trick is to revisit situations in the past where you achieved certain goals through physical exertion. Do you have any such memories that you can tap into? For example, if you were ever a part of a sports team back in school, try to remember scenarios where you really had to exert yourself to accomplish some sort of victory. Remember how difficult it was for you to do it. Remember how much you were tempted to quit. Remember how hard you fought the urge to quit. Finally, remember how happy you were when you won. If you don't have an athletic history to tap into, you can try using memories of other types of hardships that turned into victories. When you remind yourself how sweet past victories were, you will feel more motivated to carry on even when things get particularly difficult. In fact, if you are really committed to this mental exercise, you may even start enjoying your pain! You will realize that with each painful stride, you are one step closer to the sweet taste of victory.

The third trick is to focus your mind on the real reasons why you are running in the first place. As you run, and as you try to push through the pain, it's natural that negative thoughts will start popping into your head. For example, you will start thinking about how sore your legs feel, and how much your chest is burning. You can push these thoughts out of your mind by focusing on the real reasons why you are running in the first place. Are you running to improve your heart's health so that you can live longer? Are you running because you want to get in shape to impress someone you like? Are you running because you are naturally competitive, and you want to show off your athleticism? It doesn't matter if your reason for running is noble or vain. The fact is that before you started running, you were convinced that the pain of running is a worthwhile tradeoff for whatever gain you were hoping for. The purpose of this mental exercise is to remind you of that conviction, to keep you moving on towards your goal.

Music has also been known to motivate people, and to make them keep on running even when they are sore and tired. Before you go running, you can create a special playlist of songs that you find particularly motivating. It could be the lyrics or the beat of the song that inspires you—it doesn't matter, as long as that is the kind of music that keeps you pumped up and inspired. You can change the type of songs that you listen to during the run depending on the goal that you are trying to achieve. If you want to run faster, upbeat songs can help you pick up your pace. If you want to run longer (for example if you are training for a marathon), you could use songs that are a bit slow paced but are nonetheless inspiring. Some people find audiobooks and podcasts helpful when running over long distances, so you can try that out for a few sessions to see if they can work for you as well.

The human mind is designed to seek rewards, so you can use that innate drive to trick your body into pushing past its boundaries. Before you start running, you should decide that at the end of the run, you will reward yourself in a very specific way. Your reward could be anything that you truly desire. Maybe it could be a cold energy drink, a refreshing bath, or a nice breakfast. When the running gets tough, you should start thinking about that reward, and you should consider the running that you are doing to be a small obstacle that you have to overcome to get to that reward. If you are running out in nature, it's possible to build rewards into the route that you are taking. For instance, if you are running up a small hill, you could think of the scenic view from the top of the hill as your reward.

Finally, to stay positive, you can seek the help of other runners. You can find a running partner to work out with, and you could turn your running sessions into little competitions to keep each other motivated. You could also join a larger group of runners and do your sessions together. It's easy to give up or to limit yourself if you are running alone, but when you have company, you will feel the urge to push yourself further because nobody wants to appear weak in front of others. If you run in a group, everyone will be trying to keep up with everyone else, and in the end, you will all make each other better runners. Remember that if you want to truly push your limits, you should run with a group that is more advanced than you, not one that is at your level.

Keep Advancing Your Routine and Making It More Challenging

To be able to push your limits, you have to constantly keep changing your definition of what your normal capability is. For example, if at the beginning you consider a normal running session for you to be 3 miles long, in the subsequent weeks, as your endurance and speed increase, you should redefine your standard running session. You cannot push yourself to keep improving if your definition of a baseline doesn't change with time. Your philosophy here should be that "today's record is tomorrow's standard."

If you want to improve as a runner, you have to keep records of your running activities. You can have a special notebook for this purpose, but these days, there are so many fitness apps in the market, and you can use one of them to keep accurate records of your running activities. Make sure that you note down the dates, the distances that you ran, and your running times. By keeping records, you will be able to tell if you are making any improvements, if you are stagnant, or if you are regressing. You will then be able to identify ways to make improvements. For example, if you notice that your speeds are lower during certain days of the week, find out why, and try to figure out a way to make your running sessions during those days more productive.

You have to create goals that are reasonable and achievable. Look at your records for the past month and find your best running time during that period. Now, in the coming weeks and months, your primary goal will be to either match or to beat that time. This is a reasonable goal for you because you know for a fact that you can run that fast, and because you understand that by exerting yourself a little harder than you have in the past, it wouldn't be too difficult for you to beat that record. Running goals don't necessarily have to be centered on timing. You can try to use other parameters to improve. For example, if you are capable of running five miles every day, you can set a new goal where you try to run the same distance, but along a route that is hillier than your regular one.

Any goal can seem insurmountable if you look at it as one large unit. So, you should shift your perspective and try to break down a long run into a series of shorter runs. For example, if you are going on a 10-mile run, you can think of it as a five-mile run, followed by a 2-mile run, then a couple of 1-mile runs, and finally, a couple of half-mile runs. You have to think of your run as a series of minor goals that you have to accomplish along the way as you move towards a much larger goal.

Mentally, this allows you to make a long run feel more manageable, but as a runner, it also helps you to strategize. For example, you could run fast during some sections and slow down to regain your breath during others. This way, you will be able to go further than you thought possible.

You can also push your limits as a runner by learning to conserve energy while you run. As you keep running, you will notice that you always hit a lag when you reach a certain point. That often means that you haven't properly regulated the way you are exerting yourself during the few minutes leading up to that point. During subsequent running sessions, when you are about to reach that lagging point, you should slow yourself down slightly but keep on running. You might be surprised to find that instead of lagging at your usual point, you are able to maintain an impressive pace for a much longer distance.

Finally, to challenge yourself, you need to switch up the conditions under which you run. For example, if you usually run in the morning, you could try running in the afternoon when it's slightly hotter outside. If you are used to running on a paved path, you could try running out there in the wilderness. It's possible to push your limit and to challenge your boundaries just by making the conditions under which you run slightly tougher.

Chapter 6: How to Select Your Running Gear

When you invest in the right kind of running gear, you will have more productive running sessions. That's because the right gear can make your runs a lot more comfortable and safer, and it can boost your athletic performance. Of all the running gear that you will purchase, your running shoes will be the most important. We will discuss in detail how to find the right running shoes, and then we will also look at how you can select other types of running gear.

Selecting the Right Running Shoes

You are more likely to get injured while running if you wear the wrong type of shoes. You should select the right shoes based on your stride. If you visit an orthopedist or if you go to a professional sportswear store, they can be able to determine what kind of shoe you need, based on how your foot either pronates or rolls in an inward direction whenever your leg hits the ground as you run. If your foot pronates too much, or if it doesn't pronate enough, you are at a greater risk of injury. The shoe you wear will be decided upon after the specialist examines your stride.

Even though there are technical aspects to selecting a perfect running shoe, there are still some things that you can figure out on your own without needing the help of a professional. For instance, you can ensure that the upper part of the shoe that you select is shaped just like your feet. That part should also be fairly smooth when you touch it. The ankle collar of your shoe (that is the upper part of the back side of the shoe) should be well padded so that it provides support at the back of your heel, and you should make sure that it doesn't expose that part of your foot to injury. The padding at the ankle collar should also be coated with soft material so that it doesn't irritate your Achilles tendon as you run.

The saddle of your shoes should also fit perfectly over your foot, and it should be able to secure the foot so that you don't feel as though it is slipping off while you are running. The toe box of your shoe shouldn't press too hard on your toes, but it should give your toes enough room to spread around and to flex in a natural way. Also, the toe box shouldn't press your toes together, either vertically or horizontally.

The outer sole of your shoe will determine how comfortable your runs will be, and how durable your shoes will be. It should be made of materials that are highly durable, preferably rubber. The material in question should also provide enough traction for you as you run.

The midsole of the shoe is the foam material that fills the gap between your outer and inner soles. In a proper running shoe, this part should be very thick, and it should have adequate shock absorbing properties. It should be thicker at the heel area than at the front part of the shoe, and it should act to increase cushioning, as well as stability.

A running shoe must have a heel to toe drop so that it can hold your weight properly and reduce the stress that occurs in the weaker parts of your foot. Finally, you need to get a lot of high-quality socks or sock liner to go with your shoes and make sure that you switch them out every day.

Other Items That You Will Need for Your Running Sessions

After you have found the right shoes, you need to find other running gear, including the clothes that you will wear, and the accessories that you will need as you run. When it comes to selecting the right clothing for your running sessions, you want to make sure that you wear clothes that are light, comfortable, and weather appropriate. You don't have to get fancy and expensive clothing items that you see in movies or in sports ads. As long as the clothing you put on is comfortable and breathable, you are good to go. Don't dress heavily when it's warm outside and don't dress lightly when it's cold outside. Try to avoid wearing pants that are too tight (unless they are breathable) because they can make you less comfortable as you run. Other than that, you can pretty much wear anything you want.

These days, there are lots of accessories that you can come in handy when you are running. Lots of runners carry heart monitors for various reasons. If it's medically important, your doctor could recommend that you carry a heart monitor with you so that you can keep track of your levels of exertion. You can also bring a heart monitor along for non-medical reasons, especially if you like to collect a lot of data on your running sessions.

You may also need a running watch. Running watches aren't that expensive, and they don't need to be fancy either. As long as you can glance at your watch occasionally and know how well you are doing in terms of timing, your watch will be serving its purpose.

Some runners like to bring along iPods or mp3 players so that they can listen to music or podcasts as they run. If you do this, make sure that you arrange to have it anchored somehow so that you won't have to hold it in your hand. Carrying objects in your hands as you run can be distracting, and it can affect your performance.

You can also wear sunglasses as you run to protect your eyes from bright lights, UV rays, or even dust. If you choose to do this, make sure that you get the kind of sports sunglasses that are strapped down so that you won't have to keep readjusting them all the time.

Thanks to new technologies, you can now take advantage of devices such as Fitbits to monitor lots of parameters that are related to your running. You might want to purchase such devices because they will make it a lot easier for you to assess your running sessions and figure out which areas need improvement.

Chapter 7: How Beginners Should Structure Hour-Long Running Session

As a beginner, before you structure your hour-long running session, you first have to assess your baseline level of fitness. Beginners vary in their running capability because they have different levels of fitness, which are determined by the kind of activities that they were doing before they picked up running. If you worked out a lot before you decided to start running, you might be able to start at a higher level compared to someone who just got off the couch for the first time.

To accommodate the varying capacities of different beginners, we will look at the hour-long training schedule that could be used by absolute beginners, and then we will examine the schedule that could be used by beginners who already have a considerable level of fitness.

Remember that these schedules aren't written in stone—they are just supposed to act as a guide for you, or some sort of framework upon which you can base your own much more customized plan. For the purposes of distinction, we will call the beginners who haven't been working out "absolute beginner." As for those who take up running when they already are a bit physically fit, we will call them "fit beginners."

Training Schedule for Absolute Beginners

You can tell that you are an absolute beginner if you aren't capable of running for ten continuous minutes, at an intermediate pace. When left to guess which type of beginners they are, many people assume that are fit beginners, because their egos don't allow them to consider the possibility that they might be absolute beginners.

We recommend that you test yourself to determine which category you fall under. Go outside or get on a treadmill and try to run at an intermediate pace for ten continuous minutes. If you can accomplish that, then you should skip this part and go to the "fit beginners" section of this chapter immediately. However, if you find that you can't run for 10 minutes, you should start with this section.

There is no shame in admitting to yourself that you are an absolute beginner. In fact, the best way for you to learn is by starting at the very bottom of the program. If you overestimate your ability and you begin with a schedule that is too advanced for you to handle, you will be stressed out the entire time, and you might be tempted to quit.

So, to help you create your own hour-long schedule here is an example of how you can structure an hour-long training session for absolute beginners:

The schedule should run for 4 weeks, and each week should have 3 training sessions. You want to space out the 3 running sessions throughout the week so that you have a day of rest between each session. As you start, you will be doing a "walk and run" plan, which involves alternating between fast-paced walking and a few minutes of running.

For the first week, you should start each session with a basic warm up. Try to do a few jumping jacks if you can and try to jog in place for a while to loosen your muscles. You should then stretch your entire body to reduce the risk of injury. That's important because injuries are very common among beginners, and it can be very disheartening if you got injured during your first week as a runner. After you are done stretching, you should start your session with a ten-minute brisk walk.

After you have been walking for ten minutes, you should jog slowly for one full minute, and then switch to walking fast for the next one minute. You should keep repeating the one minute of walking and the one minute of jogging in alternating order for most of the remainder of your session until you have to cool down.

We expect that your warm-up will take five minutes, your stretching will take ten minutes, and the remainder of your "run and walk" session should take about 45 minutes. You should spare the last five minutes of that 45 minutes for a cool down because, again, you want to reduce your risk of injury. When you jog for one minute and walk for the next minute, the one minute of jogging will be your workout, and the minute of walking will be a rest (although, given the fast pace of the walk, it will serve to keep your heart rate up without tiring you out). The point of this type of scheduling is to take advantage of the interval training model.

During the second week of training, do your warm-up and stretching as usual, and then start out with a ten-minute walk just like you did in the first week. However, when you get to the jogging part, this time you should do it at 2-minute intervals. Run at a slow pace for 2 minutes, then walk at a fast pace for the next 2 minutes. You should keep repeating the 2-minute intervals until you are either burned out or until you are finished with your workout. You should remember to spare the 5 minutes at the end of your training session for the cool down.

During the third week, you should do pretty much the same thing where the warm-up, stretching, and cool down are concerned. However, you should switch your jogging to 3 minutes, while keeping your walking breaks at 2 minutes. The point of this is to spend more time jogging and less time walking on an incremental basis. Since you are at the infancy of your running training, you just have to go as far as you can, and it's okay if you aren't able to finish the sessions at first.

During the fourth week, everything that you will do prior to and after the running stays the same but you should shift your intervals to 5 minutes for the jogging and 2 minutes for the walking. As you improve, you should keep going on with the same pattern to see how far you can get. In the end, your ultimate aim will be to run for the whole period of time with only a single 2-minute walking break in the middle of the running session.

Once you are finished with the first four weeks of training, you should carry on with the rest of the sessions, following the same procedure. When you get to the final session of this training program (i.e. the one with a single walking break), you should do that session for one week, and then in the weeks after that, you should try to increase your jogging pace continuously.

Finally, as you get even more comfortable, get rid of that 2-minute break and run for an entire 30 minutes without having to stop. In that case, your session will be a five-minute warm-up, ten minutes of stretching, ten minutes of walking, 30 minutes of jogging, and a 5-minute cool down. If you can do this comfortably, your training as an absolute beginner will be complete, and you can now graduate into the fit beginner category.

Training Schedule for Fit Beginners

If you have been working out in other ways, and if you have a considerable level of fitness, to begin with, you might be able to start running at a more advanced level than absolute beginners, so your running schedule could stand to be more rigorous than that of someone who hasn't been working out at all.

Perhaps you have been doing some strength training at the gym, and you have built up some considerable level of endurance. Perhaps you have been cycling during the evenings and weekends, so your leg muscles are fairly developed. Perhaps you have been swimming for fun several times a week, so your cardiovascular system is strong. Whatever physical activity you were involved in, you could be fit enough to skip the "absolute beginner" course. You should take the 10-minute running test to see if you are already capable of handling yourself. If you can run for ten minutes at an intermediate pace without completely burning out, then you are qualified to train under the fit beginner schedule.

Just like the program for absolute beginners, this one also involves both running and walking, but because it's more intensive, it also includes periods of rest. The rest periods are necessary to lower the risk of injury and to reduce fatigue as well as stress. In this program, you will be training for 6 out of 7 days every week, and you will be taking one day to recover. However, it's important to note that not all workout sessions will involve running. In fact, at the beginning of the program, there are days when all you have to do is just walk.

During the first week, you should start your hour-long training session on the first day with a five to ten-minute warm-up, then you should spend ten more minutes stretching. Once you are done stretching, you should run for thirty minutes. For the first week, it's okay to jog slowly for the entire 30 minutes. You may only walk for a couple of minutes, right in the middle of your run (starting on the 14-minute mark). However, it's preferable to push through all the way to the end of the 30 minutes, even if you have to do it at a slow pace.
On the second day of the first week, you should start with the warm up and you should stretch as usual, but then you should walk for the remainder of the one-hour session. You will notice that compared to the

program for absolute beginners, instead of skipping one day between running sessions, fit beginners have to walk during those days. For the rest of the first week, you should do the running and the walking session in alternating order, except for the one day when you have to take a rest.

Your second week of training will be exactly the same as the first week, except for the fact that you can try to increase your running pace if you feel more comfortable with it. However, during the third week of your training, you should start introducing an element of distance into your hour-long running schedule. Instead of just running for a specific period of time (in many cases 30 minutes), you should try to run for a specific distance. For example, instead of jogging for 30 minutes, try to jog for 2 miles.

As you begin to incorporate this change into your running schedule, you may realize that at first, you will be spending more time running than the one hour that you have allocated to each session. If you have a busy schedule after your running session, you could cut it short and keep a record of how much distance you were unable to cover. Keep trying to increase your pace with every subsequent session, until you are able to cover the requisite distance within your workout session. If your calendar is open for the hours after your running session, you could add a few minutes to your session and try to cover the remainder of the distance. As a runner, you have to build both your speed and your endurance, so you shouldn't only focus on one of those aspects.

To make your hour-long training schedule more meaningful, you could set an objective that you have to achieve when you finish your training program. For example, you could decide to sign up for a 5K-race 3 months after you start your first training session, and you could work progressively to build your capacity as a runner so that you would be able to accomplish that goal. In fact, many beginners have found that training towards a specific goal keeps them more motivated and focused, and it increases their odds of becoming great runners.

You should use either of the schedules we have discussed here to structure your own hour-long training sessions. You know yourself better than anyone else, and you know what goals you have in mind as a runner, so nobody is better placed to design a beginner running program for you. Just make sure that the program you create has incremental levels of difficulty, and that as you follow it, you keep pushing and challenging yourself to be a better runner.

Chapter 8: Dietary Requirements for Novice Joggers

As a runner, you need to remember that proper nutrition is extremely important given the fact that you will be constantly engaging in physically strenuous activities. That means that you need to carefully consider what effect each food item that you include in your diet is going to have on your body. In this chapter, we discuss the dietary requirements that all beginner runners need to keep in mind.

What You Should Eat Before Running

You need to fuel your body properly before you go out on a run. Basically, you need to top up your body's glycogen reserves so that you have enough energy for your run. The kind of food you should eat before the run depends on the distance that you are planning to cover during that day's session. If you intend to go on a short run, eating beforehand isn't really that crucial. However, if you intend to go on a prolonged running session, you might want to ensure that you have the energy reserves you need to cover that distance.

If you go on an intensive long distance run on an empty stomach, it could have a net negative effect on your fitness, because your body might start breaking down muscle in order to create the energy that you need to spend during that exercise. Prior to a short run, you can just grab a fruit on your way out. Having a banana, an apple, or a handful of grapes can be enough to give you an energy boost for a short run. If you don't want to eat fruit, you can have a healthy snack before the short run. A piece of toast or a single muffin will be enough. Alternatively, you could also eat one half of an energy bar to get that energy boost.

If you are going on a longer run, it's important to fill up on carbohydrate-rich foods because such running sessions tend to burn a lot of energy. However, make sure that you eat complex carbohydrates, and not simple ones. Common sources of complex carbs include whole wheat foods, oatmeal etc. You want to make sure that you eat foods that aren't too refined because the refining process tends to get rid of fiber. You need fiber-rich foods for long distance runs because fiber tends to break down much slower, which means that the glucose from the food will be released into your bloodstream at a slow but constant rate, and this will give you enough energy to sustain you for the duration of the run.

You should also add a little bit of protein and healthy fats into your pre-workout meal. They will help you feel fuller and therefore more comfortable during your run. However, don't do it excessively, because these two food types tend to break down quite slowly, and they won't be of much help for you during your running session (in terms of providing an energy boost). In fact, if you eat a lot of fatty foods before you go running, you could get stomach upsets, and this could affect your performance out there.

Finally, if you are eating before you go on a run, make sure that you do it one hour or at least a half an hour before you actually start your exercise. This will give your body the time it needs to start digesting that food. If you eat just before you go for a run, your body will redirect large volumes of blood towards the intestines to aid with the digestion process, and this will affect your performance as a runner.

Should You Eat or Drink While Running?

If you are running over a short distance, there is absolutely no need to eat or drink anything during the run. However, if you are having a long-running session, you might want to have a plan on how to stay energized and well hydrated throughout the session. You can carry a water bottle in a backpack so that you can take sips of water as you run out in nature. If you feel the need, you can dilute some glucose in the water beforehand so that it can give you a little extra energy during your long-distance run. Alternatively, you can bring a bottle of a drink that is rich in electrolytes if you don't want to drink water. Some runners bring various types of soft candy with them on the run, but if you do this, you should be careful not to overindulge.

What to Eat After Running

After you have finished your running session, you should eat foods that help you recover from the run. Whatever meal you choose, make sure that it has some carbs and some protein in it. Carbs will help to refill your glycogen stores, which will be depleted, especially if you have just finished a long-distance running session. Carbs are digested rather quickly, so they'll help refill your energy reserves much faster. Protein, on the other hand, will help to repair any muscles that may have been damaged or distressed during the run.

What to Include in Your Diet During the Training Period

Once you have begun training, you need to make sure that you eat a well-balanced diet every single day. You should also make sure that you have all your meals, and that you don't skip any of them. You want to be able to keep your strength up at all times, not just when you are about to go out for a run. That's because the running process causes a lot of distress to the body, and your muscles are always in repair mode all around the clock, so you need to provide them with the nutrients that they need to repair and to grow. In order to make sure that your diet is well balanced, you should always plan your meals beforehand. It's okay to take supplements if you feel that there are nutrients of which you aren't getting enough from your diet but remember that it's always better to source all your nutrients from real foods.

Chapter 9: How to Become the Best Runner That You Can Be

To become the best runner that you can be, you have to continuously improve in all area, including your speed, your discipline, your endurance, and your efficiency. Ultimately, it's not about being faster than other people; it really is about achieving your peak potential as a runner and living with the knowledge that every time you put on those running shoes, and you will be giving it 100%. Here are important tips you should follow if you want to become the best runner that you can be:

Study More Experienced Runners

You can't be your best self as a runner if you don't take the time to learn how to do it correctly, and one of the best ways for you to learn how to run is by studying accomplished runners. Is there a professional runner that you consider to be your role model?

Of course, you are not trying to get into the Olympics, but you still can learn a lot from those who are the best at running. If you want to be better at long distance running, look for tapes of marathon winner and listen to what they say about how hard they work, where they find motivation, and what they consider to be their secrets to success.

You can also watch tapes of races, preferably those with commentaries from professional coaches, to learn about the best techniques that are used by runners at a professional level. If you keep tabs on athletes who manage to accomplish great things on the track, your practice sessions won't feel so unbearable anymore, and you will start believing that you too can be much better than you initially thought. That belief can motivate you and propel you to new heights.

Be Disciplined and Deliberate in Your Practice

To be the best runner that you can be, you have to be disciplined, and you must be very deliberate in your practice. You should make a practice schedule, and you should follow it religiously. No matter what comes up, do not skip your running sessions. In fact, the only thing that should keep you away from running should be an injury (and even then, you shouldn't take too many days off).

You should also prepare yourself psychologically to run under difficult circumstances. If it rains during your workout time, that is not an excuse to skip it. Put on a raincoat and hit the pavement. You will feel an even greater sense of accomplishment after that session. If you have to travel to another city for work, or if you have to go away on vacation, that is no reason to skip running sessions. Make sure you pack your running shoes and try to look up some of the best running routes when you get to your destination. You will be surprised to realize that you are more motivated to run because of the change of scenery.

Sign Up for Competitions

The best way to know if you are close to your real potential as a runner is by signing up to compete in a few races. Usually, you can sign up for a race a few months before the actual event, and you can restructure your running sessions and turn them into practice sessions for the upcoming race. If you started out as a beginner, and you have been running for a while, you can try to test your new abilities as a runner by signing up for a 5K race. If you are a bit more advanced, you can sign up for a 10K or even a much longer race. You don't sign up for these races because you are trying to win, you do it because you just want to have that sense of accomplishment when you finally cross the finish line. If you indeed do participate in a race and you complete it, you will be more confident and more motivated as a runner.

Try Speed Exercises

If you have been improving in terms of the distance that you cover during the running sessions, you can become better by switching things up once in a while and trying speed exercises. If you live in an area with hilly terrain, try sprinting up the hill as you time yourself. Do this at least once every week. With every subsequent attempt, your goal should be to beat your previous record. You should also try running on an actual track and timing yourself. As a runner, it's important to keep challenging your own best times.

You should know how fast you can run a single lap around the track, how long it would take you to run a single mile, or how fast your 100-meter sprint is. One way to make yourself a faster runner is by trying to run with a tempo. The best way to do this is by using an upbeat song to set that tempo. Play a fast song on your iPod and try to run to the beat of that song for as long as you can. The more you practice, the more your speed will improve.

Increase Your Practice Time as You Gain Experience

If you started out with hour-long running sessions, and you find that you are comfortable running for the entire time while covering a considerable distance, you should step things up by increasing your practice time. If you keep growing as a runner, you will eventually outgrow the one-hour session, and you will need more time per session to really push your limits. If you can't find extra time during the week, you can try to lengthen your sessions during the weekend so that you can really be able to explore the outer limits of your running capabilities.

Chapter 10: Injury Avoidance and Recovery Techniques That Every Runner Should Know

Being a physical activity, running is inherently dangerous, and so when you take it up, you should do everything in your power to protect yourself from injuries. However, despite your best efforts, you might still get injured as a result of running. This shouldn't discourage you from becoming a runner. The benefits of running outweigh the risks by far, so running is still worth it for you. In this chapter, we discuss the steps that you can take to avoid injury, and in case you still get injured after taking all the precautions, we will follow up with techniques on how to recover from injury.

How to Prevent Injuries

Most running-related injuries come from issues with flexibility. To increase your flexibility before you go out on a run, you need to stretch. In fact, it's necessary to stretch on a daily basis, not just to prevent injury, but also to improve your performance. When you start your exercise routine, your first activity should be a warm-up, then it should be followed by stretching. When you stretch, you have to follow the right technique. First, you have to avoid rushing through the stretching session. You should hold every position that you take during your stretch for at least 30 seconds without moving around.

You also need to warm up before you start running, and you need to cool down after you are done running. Warm-ups are supposed to precede stretching sessions (although it's okay to mix up with two). Your warm-up sessions should depend on the kind of running exercise that you intend to perform. If you want to run fast, you need to warm up for much longer. When you warm up, you are essentially flushing out wastes such as lactic acid from your muscles, and this reduces the chances of experiencing muscle soreness.

One of the main reasons why people get injured while running is because they lack the strength and stamina to run for sustained periods of time. In other words, beginners may get injured because they aren't athletic enough. To rectify this, you need to supplement your running with some strength training. You need to build some muscle and to improve your general level of athleticism in order to make yourself less prone to injuries. Unless you bring up your general physical strength, your muscles will get tired pretty fast, and the end result will be a high susceptibility to injuries, and longer recovery time in the event that the injuries actually occur. You could try to lift some weights to build your upper body strength. It's also possible to increase muscle strength by running along routes that are challenging.

You can also reduce your chances of injury by drinking more fluids. If you run while you are not properly hydrated, you run the risk of experiencing heat exhaustion. It's advisable to drink water roughly two hours before your running session to make sure that you are well hydrated the moment you start running. As you run, you should carry some water with you so that you can drink about 7 ounces of it after every 15 minutes or so. Also, make sure that you drink a lot of water a couple of hours after your exercise. As you drink water, you may also need an energy boost, so you can dilute some glucose in your water to form a carbohydrate solution. If you have access to energy drinks that are rich in electrolytes, you can substitute them for water (you should, however, be careful when choosing energy drinks since some of them are full of empty calories, which could negate your entire reason for exercising in the first place).

You should include resting days in your training schedule. Even though you are trying to maximize the health and fitness benefits of your running session, it's unwise to do it every single day because this increases your chances of getting injured. When you take up running, your body would need some time to adapt to the activity, so it would be better for you to skip some days to let the body recover from exposure to intense activities. If you still feel the need to work out during the off days, you could try other fitness activities such as weight training.

You should also increase your running distance in a slow progression so that your body can be able to handle the stress much better. If you take on intensive exercises in quick progression, your chances of getting injured will go through the roof. What you need to do is to start small, and then increase the intensity of your running sessions as the body adjusts. Most fitness experts recommend that the duration, the amount, and the difficulty of the running exercises that you perform should be increased by about 7% every week (but it should be kept at the same level for the duration of the week, not bumped up by a percentage point each day).

You can also reduce your chances of getting injured by having the right type of running gear. That means that you should run in the right type of shoes. There are different types of shoes available for people with different shapes of feet as well as styles of running, so make sure that you know what category you fall under. If you go to a sports store that sells footwear for athletes, they'll be able to examine your feet and tell you exactly what kind of shoes you need to protect yourself from injuries.

Some people work out their glutes to reduce their chances of getting injured. Others foam-roll their thighs and calves to achieve the same goal. Still, others work out their cores to increase their general levels of stability, thus reducing the chances of injury. If you are considering these and other options that we haven't mentioned here, that is okay, as long as you remember to confirm that the science behind your injury prevention method is really sound.

Finally, to prevent injuries, you need to listen to your body. Throughout the book, we have encouraged you to push through the pain when you are running so as to extend your limit, but here we are going to tell you to learn the difference between soreness due to physical exertion, and the kind of pain that indicates that you have on an oncoming injury. If you feel as though you are about to develop an injury, you should see your doctor to confirm your suspicion, and you should follow the instructions that the doctor gives you in order to prevent the injury.

How to Recover from Injuries

Unfortunately, you may still get injured even after taking all the necessary precautions. When this happens, it's going to be a painful experience, and you are going to get a bit frustrated, particularly if you had a major upcoming racing event that you were preparing for. However, you shouldn't be afraid to take time off to recover from your injury. Sometimes, if you decide to push through the injury, it could make everything so much worse. Taking time off doesn't mean that you have failed as a runner, it just means that you have the good sense not to worsen an injury.

You should remember that the longer the recovery period, the more ground you lose, so you should try to act quickly by using home remedies to soothe your injury. However, if the pain persists, don't hesitate to see a physical therapist.

As you take a break from running to recover from an injury, you could keep up your fitness levels by doing some cross training. You can also consult your physical therapist, and he could recommend activities that you could do without causing your injury to flare up. If your caregiver gives you the clearance, it might be possible to replace running with other cardio activities such as riding a bike or swimming. If you are training as a runner, one of the best activities for you as you recover from the injury would be "aqua jogging." This term refers to an exercise where participants "jog" while underwater. With such exercises, won't apply enough pressure on the leg to agitate the injury, but you will be able to put in the hours of exercise that you need to maintain your current level of fitness.

The "runner's knee" is one of the most common injuries that you can encounter as a jogger. The injury often affects professional athletes whose sports require a lot of running, and it's also common for non-athletes who take up running for the purposes of health and fitness. Researchers have found that this condition accountant for way over a half of all cases of knee injuries in runners. If you experience this type of injury, your best course of action would be to schedule an appointment with your physiotherapist to try and find out the extent of the injury. You can be able to tell if you have the runner's knee if you feel twinges of pain, either outside or inside the knee as you start your running session. You may feel okay as you carry on with the session, but after you are finished, the pain will flare up again. The pain could come back when you least expect it, especially if you sit down for long periods of time. When this happens, you would know that the problem is getting a lot worse, and you would be well advised to seek medical attention.

You may also experience injuries that are related to the hamstrings. Injuries related to hamstrings often arise because of issues with either strength or flexibility, so you may be able to avoid such injuries by doing some strength training or by stretching the muscle before you go running. Hamstrings make up most of the muscles at the back part of your thighs, and these muscles are responsible for propulsion in the running process. Hamstring injuries may be able to heal on their own, but they take a lot of time to do so. We recommend resting for a while and doing other physical activities as you allow the injury to heal. However, you should be careful, and you should take note of the extent of the injury so that you can be able to tell if you actually need professional medical attention. If you feel a constant tightness or an ache in the back of your legs while running, and you are forced to slow down your pace in an attempt to ease your pain, then you are dealing with a hamstring-related injury. You should see a physiotherapist as soon as possible before the problem becomes magnified.

Another common injury that runners experience is the one related to the Achilles tendon. This tendon links the major muscles in your calf to the back part of your heel. If the tendon gets a bit irritated, or if it tightens unexpectedly, it could cause a lot of pain in the back of the foot. The best recovery technique for someone experiencing "Achilles tendinitis" is to apply ice to the affected area, and let it rest for a while. This often works to sooth the pain, and for most people, it's often enough. However, if the pain keeps coming back even when you aren't running at the time, then you should seriously consider seeing a physiotherapist.

You may also experience running injuries that are referred to as "plantar fasciitis." These types of injuries involve slight tears and a bit of inflammation on the ligaments and the tendons within the foot. The injuries often present in form of dull pain accompanied by bruises on either the heels or the arches of your feet. Resting may ease the pain from such an injury, but you should monitor it to tell if it's escalating. If you experience pain in your feet early in the morning as you get off the bed, you should know that it's time to see a physiotherapist.

You might also experience injuries due to conditions such as IT band syndrome, shin splints, and stress fractures, for all these injuries, ice can be a great remedy to sooth the pain temporarily, but in all cases, you must seek medical attention if the pain doesn't seem to decline at least a few hours after you are done with your running session.

Conclusion

Thank you for making it through to the end of *The Novice Runner's Handbook: A Comprehensive Guide to Get You Started as a Runner or Jogger*. Let us hope that the knowledge that you have gained from reading this book will provide you with the necessary tools to become an excellent runner or jogger, and it will help you achieve all your fitness goals.

The next step is to get out there and start running. It's going to be difficult at first, but you should work hard to push through that initial hesitation. Once you learn to push yourself hard and to overcome the pain using the tricks that you have learned in this book, you will start to see the benefits of running, and you will start reaping the fruits of your labor.

The greatest runners in the world started somewhere. So, if you are a beginner today and if you are struggling to find the motivation and the strength to get started, you shouldn't despair. No matter how challenging things get, you should know that the pain and the difficulty are what bring forth all the benefits that you have read about in this book. You have seen that your life can be transformed through running, and you have discovered that running could also preserve your health or even save your life. When the going gets tough, you shouldn't lose sight of why you are running in the first place and what it is that you are working towards.

You should also remember to keep growing as a runner. Don't stay stagnant. If you have achieved a certain fitness goal through running, don't think that it's the end of it. You should set new goals and start to work towards them. Every day, you should work towards beating your own records. Try to run faster, try to run longer. Don't ever stop growing and improving.

As you transform your life through running or jogging, don't do it alone. You should try to bring others along with you through that transformation. If you have friends who you think could benefit from taking up jogging, teach them what you know and try to work with them and help them get to where you are. You have learned in the book that when you run with others, you can challenge each other, and you can all become better runners.

Running is a fun activity, and the more you do it, the better you will learn to enjoy it. Even if you are not an Olympic gold medalist, you should learn to cherish all your accomplishments as a runner.

www.ingramcontent.com/pod-product-compliance
Lightning Source LLC
Chambersburg PA
CBHW051352280526
45784CB00007B/2922